Changing Hospital Environments for Children

This volume is published as part of a long-standing cooperative program between the Harvard University Press and the Commonwealth Fund, a philanthropic foundation, to encourage the publication of significant scholarly books in medicine and health.

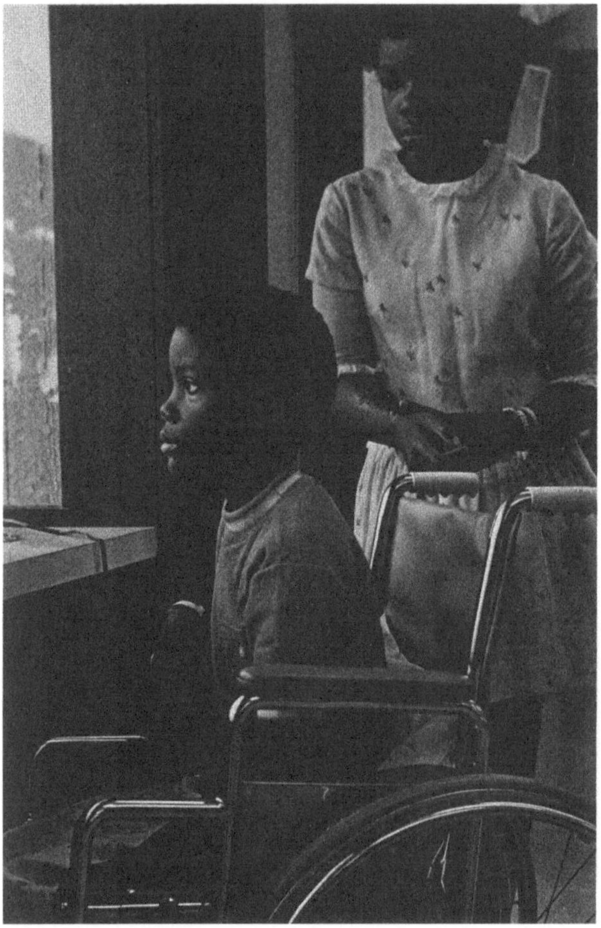

# Changing Hospital Environments for Children

Roslyn Lindheim, Helen H. Glaser, and Christie Coffin

*Photographs by Lise Giødesen*

*A Commonwealth Fund Book*
Harvard University Press, Cambridge, Massachusetts, 1972

Printed in the United States of America
Library of Congress Catalog Number 75–188969
SBN 674–10825–6

To the children and staff of
Children's Hospital at Stanford

# Foreword

The medical and architectural literature has long lacked any serious study of the physical environment of a hospital for children, and of that environment's relation to and impact on the total, critical milieu surrounding the child, including its medical, psychological, social, recreational, and educational aspects. This unique book fills that gap. It offers a comprehensive review of the world's literature on the hospitalized child, effectively organized in a developmental sequence that recognizes the distinctive characteristics of various age groupings.

Having worked personally with the senior authors in the design and implementation of programs in the new Children's Hospital at Stanford, I know first hand of their expertise in and dedication to the development of optimum hospital environments for children. When in 1964 the hospital reached the decision to rebuild, a process of planning and design began that was to culminate five years later in the completion of an entirely new physical plant and outside environs. Not often has a facility been given the opportunity literally to start from scratch. Roslyn Lindheim, who was hired as a consulting architect for programming and research, began the painstaking task of defining the principles that should be followed in construction of a positive hospital environment for children. Considerable efforts were made to include all users of the hospital in the decision-making process. Consultation with the entire staff, from doctors to janitors, occurred at many points in the design process.

After extensive observations and interviews, Professor Lindheim prepared a tentative program incorporating the ideas of the staff. This program was carefully reviewed by all personnel; concepts were clarified, many points changed, and a new program was developed. The staff then met away from the hospital for several days to finalize their ideas. This interchange provided an opportunity for each group of users to understand better the needs of the others. Those features of design that were ultimately judged essential to meeting our needs were incorporated in the facility by the architectural firm of Stone, Marraccini, and Patterson.

Professor Lindheim has subsequently met with the hospital staff on an ongoing basis to maintain a continuing evaluation of the interaction between the physical environment and those who use it. Members of the staff who were involved in the planning and design process and thus had a commitment to the result have been more satisfied with the building than have those who started to work in the hospital after the design was complete. Moreover, despite efforts to include all users, some were left out — namely house officers and parents — and the design suffered as a result because sufficient facilities for these groups were not included. It is clear that measures to include all hospital users in the planning process are essential to a successful project.

In 1965 Dr. Helen H. Glaser, a pediatrician with a deep interest in the developmental and behavioral aspects of both the well and the sick child, who later entered psychiatry, joined the hospital's medical staff as assistant medical director. At that time the design of the new hospital had been completed, but construction had not yet begun. Having worked in the old buildings and then participated in the process of adapting patient care activities to the newly completed facilities, in whose design she had no part, she was able to bring an objective point of view to the evolution of the new environment. Dr. Glaser met frequently with all members of the staff and was aware of and concerned with every facet of the hospital, from food service to accommodations for visiting parents. Her knowledge of the psychological as well as medical needs of children of all ages made her particularly sensitive to the fit between the environment and the needs of children in different age groups.

It was during the process of evaluating the new hospital that the idea of this book was first conceived by Professor Lindheim and Dr. Glaser. In 1969 they started writing, aided by a grant from the San Francisco Foundation and the Commonwealth Fund. They were subsequently joined by Christie Coffin, an architect who has in recent years devoted her professional efforts to exploring the social and behavioral aspects of architecture. Recognizing the need to link principles of child growth and development to concepts of physical design in hospital planning, the authors drew heavily on their observations of patterns of patient care at the Children's Hospital at Stanford, both before and after construction of the new facility. Their goal was to make these observations and the implications generally available to child health professionals and hospital planners. It is gratifying to know that what was learned from the errors will help future planners and designers of children's facilities to do an even better job.

The many illustrations used in the text highlight both the best features of the new hospital and its mistakes. They reflect the sensitivity of the photographer, Lise Giødesen, an occupational therapist at the hospital who was able, through her familiarity with the setting, to capture the essence of hospital life in its natural state.

Readers of this book will find that the theories of child development and behavior which underlie the design recommendations are fully documented. At the same time, the "how to's" of design are concise, clearly thought out, and understandable to any person interested in children's hospital design. The product of a rare combination of experience and interprofessional background, this book meets an important need for authoritative information and guidance on hospital design for children. More important, it should in future greatly enhance the ability of hospitals to provide better care for children and their families when faced with the stress of illness and hospitalization.

M. Harry Jennison, M.D.
Executive Director
Children's Hospital at Stanford

# Acknowledgments

We cannot hope to mention personally the many architects, physicians, nurses, therapists, psychologists, teachers, child care workers, volunteers, parents, and of course children with whom we talked and who gave freely of their time and advice to make this book possible. We would especially like to thank the staff, children, and families of Children's Hospital at Stanford, Palo Alto, California, to whom this book is dedicated, and without whose active participation the many fine photographs by Lise Giødesen would not have been possible.

We are deeply grateful to a number of other hospitals for opening their facilities to our observation and freeing staff time for consultation. These include Stanford University Medical Center; Children's Hospital of Los Angeles; Children's Hospital, San Francisco; Colorado General Hospital, Denver; Greater Baltimore Medical Center; Johns Hopkins Children's Medical and Surgical Center, Baltimore; Kaiser Foundation Hospital, Oakland; Mt. Zion Hospital, San Francisco; Shriners Hospital for Crippled Children, San Francisco; St. Luke's Hospital, St. Paul, Minnesota; St. Mary's Hospital and Medical Center, San Francisco; and Wyler Children's Hospital, Chicago.

We are indebted to our numerous friends and colleagues for their help in the preparation of the manuscript. We particularly thank Emma N. Plank, Cleveland Metropolitan General Hospital; Robert J. Haggerty, University of Rochester Medical School; Carl Eisdorfer, Duke University Medical Center; Bertrand Goldberg, Marina City, Chicago; Howard A. Friedman, San Francisco; Paul Rousseau, Kaiser Foundation Hospital, Oakland; Harold R. Novotny, Palo Alto; Lucy Muldrow and Ida Castillo, Berkeley Health Department; and Fred Osmon, Berkeley. We should also like to express appreciation to Jacqueline Vischer and Stuart Sidells for research assistance; to Marvin Roos and Tom Sueoka for making prints of the photographs; to Peggie Spaulding for administering the Commonwealth Fund grant; to Elizabeth Bagwell for editorial assistance; and to Pat Miller, Sylvia Russell, Jean Blanchard, and Carolyn Linstroth for typing innumerable drafts of the manuscript.

Finally, we are grateful to our husbands, Richard Lindheim, Robert J. Glaser, and Stephen Coffin, for their expert counsel, critical review, and patient support.

R. L.
H. G.
C. C.

# Contents

# Architectural Plans

Changing Hospital Environments for Children

# Introduction

**All children should be tirelessly noisy,
playful, grubby-handed except at meal times,
soiling and tearing such clothes as they need
to wear, bringing not only the joy of childhood
into the house but the dust and mud as well;
in short, everything that makes the quiet and
order of sickness and nursing impossible.**
— George Bernard Shaw

Many children, particularly younger ones, experience ill effects from being hospitalized. The syndrome called institutionalism can smother the distinctive style and individual pattern of growth of almost any child. For example, the child who reacts against the institutionalism of the school does not learn; the child who reacts against the institutionalism of the orphanage does not develop the equivalent capabilities of a child reared at home. As an institution, however, the hospital has been particularly immune to attack on these grounds, because everything that takes place there is done from medical necessity. Yet in the hospital the child who reacts against institutionalism manifests developmental retardation, worsening medical conditions, a reversal to infantile practices, or problems with his family that may persist after his return home.

Whether in the hospital because of a hernia, acute asthma, or a congenital disorder, the child is still a baby, a four-year-old, a school-age child or a teenager — with all the needs, fears, and desires of these diverse age groups, but whose developmental needs are complicated by his simultaneous illness. Only since the sixties have pediatricians, psychiatrists, and psychologists shown that expert medical care must be supplemented by attention to a child's social, emotional, and developmental needs. It is our contention that some of the variety and richness of experience so necessary for childhood development can be accommodated within hospital walls, and is as viable for the acutely ill as for those in a convalescent stage.

In this book we attempt to develop design guidelines that can be of help in generating environments sympathetic to the needs of children of different ages who are required to live away from home for medical reasons. Alternatives to hospitalization are first explored. Where these are lacking, ways to bridge the gap between the community and the hospital are identified. The specific developmental needs of infants, toddlers and preschoolers, school-age children, and adolescents are then discussed in relation to their environmental needs, and on this basis design guidelines for hospitals are drawn up. The needs of parents and staff in the hospital environment are also examined, with particular emphasis placed on nursing unit design.

Not included is a discussion of the specialized environments required for such cases as the child in isolation, the child attached to machines — as in kidney dialysis — the child in intensive care, or the dying child, because these problems require a creative individual approach and an up-to-date knowledge of the rapidly changing technology.

# Alternatives to Hospitalization 1

Although the organization and design of environments for sick children away from home is our primary concern, it should be emphasized that institutionalization can seldom be a totally positive experience for a child and should be avoided in cases where alternatives exist. The first step, then, toward improving the overall physical and social environment of the sick child, and toward closing the gap between the potential for medical care and the actual rendering of medical services, is to seek alternatives to hospitalization. Such alternatives must include elimination of some of the situations that create the need to hospitalize children. Attention should be given to providing the social and physical environment necessary for a healthy life, as well as to providing comprehensive medical service where it is needed most and to those who need it most.

Several distinguished health professionals elaborated this point at the 1970 Conference on Health Services for Children and Youth. Speaking before the group, Robert J. Haggerty commented that the essential ingredients for good health are "good housing, safe transportation, clean air and water, noise abatement, economic conditions that provide adequate nutrition, clothing, and leisure; critical, too, are legal and social systems in which human beings are able to interact with dignity and freedom and — for children — the family and the educational environment." [1]

René Dubos has also expressed the deeply-felt conviction that "the extent of health improvements that issue from building ultra-modern hospitals with up-to-date equipment is probably trivial in comparison with the results that can be achieved at much lower cost by providing all infants and children with well-balanced food, sanitary conditions, and a stimulating environment. Needless to say, acceptance of this thesis would imply profound changes in medicosocial policies and would affect the selection of problems in scientific research." [2]

Examples of research activities that are directed toward understanding the effect of the social environment on child health are the studies of childhood injuries which show that accidents and injuries among children usually involve social situations and failures in parental coping behavior.[3]

Children's emergency hospital admissions have even been found to be significantly associated with such factors as the mother's menstruation.[4]

Similarly, hospitalization occasionally reflects the physician's own anxiety and inability to cope with a stressful situation, be it the complexity of the child's illness or of the family interaction. Assistance to the doctor in handling the social and emotional stresses related to a child's illness might sometimes obviate his need to use the hospital as a means of nonmedical crisis intervention.

Furthermore, physicians today know how to prevent the crippling effects of many diseases, as well as how to treat these diseases effectively while the patient is still ambulant. However, the ratio of physicians serving children to the child population has been dropping steadily, and the consequences of a decreased availability of pediatric care bode ill for child health in the United States.

Finally, nonwhite minorities suffer from an infant mortality rate double that of the white population — a difference that primarily reflects the low socioeconomic status of nonwhites. Poverty is four times more common for nonwhite children.[5] The preventive, diagnostic, and treatment services available to children in the United States are obviously very uneven and vary with a family's financial position: "It is perfectly clear that children and youth born into different social, cultural, or economic circumstances in the U.S. do not receive uniform attention to their medical and dental health. Those at greatest risk, with the greatest need and the least health services, are the nonwhite, the poor, the central city or rural dweller."[6]

It is of the utmost importance, therefore, to the welfare and health of children that preventive, diagnostic, therapeutic, and rehabilitative medical facilities be easily available for all children, regardless of income, ethnic group, social status, or location. Moreover, new institutional forms must be developed to accommodate the changing needs of medical treatment. Such a change would involve not only a major re-working of the existing health care system but also a significant reordering of all national priorities.

## Provide Accessibility and Familiarity

Until recent times medical admissions of children to the hospital were directed toward the treatment of infectious diseases and nutritional deficiencies. Now, congenital malformations, birth injuries, accidents, diabetes, nephrosis, asthma, cystic fibrosis, and heart disease prevail.[7] The treatment for these conditions requires increasingly sophisticated diagnostic procedures and medical and surgical techniques, particularly for very ill children. At the same time, there are now greater possibilities for evaluating and treating these conditions while the patient is still ambulant.[8]

For many afflictions, successful treatment is predicated on early diagnosis and prompt medical treatment as a means of minimizing chronic complications. Provision of mechanisms for routine preventive and diagnostic medical examinations as well as the ready availability of medical treatment services would help to accomplish this aim. Upper and middle income families meet this need by taking their children to private or group-practice pediatric offices for regular checkups or preventive care. Persons in the lower income group use the outpatient clinics and emergency departments of urban hospitals as their doctors' offices. Mothers and children crowd the emergency clinics of urban hospitals — particularly at night, when their husbands can babysit for the other children or provide necessary transportation to the hospital.

These places are often both dismal and fearful. Characteristic of the outpatient departments of many urban hospitals are the large waiting rooms with dull colored walls, the long rows of uncomfortable benches, and combined outpatient and emergency entrances through which come both the child with a sore throat and the man bleeding from a gunshot wound. Families customarily wait interminably before seeing a doctor. The waiting room and halls in emergency departments are often full of policemen, who may arouse apprehension or hostility, particularly among people of lower socioeconomic groups.

The appearance of the hospital is particularly unpleasant for children. The scale is generally large and frightening. The sight of people on gurneys and of the complicated apparatus required for treatment terrifies both the very young and the adolescent. The location of large medical centers generally requires a long, uncomfortable ride on public transit, which represents a negative reinforcement to use of the facilities for ambulant care. Although hospital-based professionals claim that the hospital is the proper institution in which to organize and implement community medical services as well as to provide in-patient care, the fact is that, "in spite of many protests to the contrary, medical centers have not done a good job of providing continuing, comprehensive services for defined population groups . . . In fact, the hospital as a major base of medical care has had an inhibiting effect on the development of community health services."[9] These difficulties are frequently compounded by severe communication problems. In bilingual communities, health workers frequently speak only English. In most communities the language of health care is the language of the middle class.

The poor are thus penalized for being sick and for being poor in the miserable health care they receive. It is little wonder that the economically disadvantaged utilize medical facilities only in time of crisis and not for prevention, diagnosis, or minor treatment. If medical facilities are to be utilized appropriately, it is essential that they be comfortable, easily accessible, appropriate to the needs of different age levels, and staffed with personnel from all subgroups within the community served.

## *Design Guidelines*

Locate preventive, diagnostic, and therapeutic ambulant facilities away from the hospital whenever medically feasible.

Locate neighborhood health stations close to where people live.[10] Ambulant services should be accessible to peoples' homes so that parents can easily bring their children, particularly infants and toddlers, for routine checkups and minor illnesses.

Staff these stations with personnel drawn from all ethnic and language groups in the neighborhood, who are familiar with other components of the health system and who can both advise parents where to go for additional services and help arrange transportation to these facilities.[11]

Provide babysitting service in each neighborhood to allow mothers to bring sick children to health facilities without neglecting siblings.

Locate medical services at every public school, and link these services to a central facility for the entire school district. Since all children from six to sixteen years of age go to school, this setting is a logical locus for broad provision of pediatric health services, whether preventive, diagnostic, or therapeutic. Various programs for screening hearing and visual defects already exist in the schools. Linking each school to a central ambulant medical center servicing a school district would guarantee every child of school age adequate medical care. Each school could contain facilities for examination and treatment of minor conditions. Children requiring more complex care or diagnosis could be brought to the school district medical center by a school health bus. Additional links between schools and the health center could be provided by computers, closed circuit TV, and other audio-visual means of communicating health records.

Provide separate facilities for teenagers. The special needs and sensibilities of teenagers must be recognized if they are to avail themselves of medical services. Adolescents appreciate separate entrances, waiting space, and services tailored to their particular problems. They need information and services pertaining to birth control, venereal disease, and drug use. They benefit from special crisis intervention services, such as the twenty-four-hour telephone "hot lines" in which sympathetic, trained listeners are on call to help handle any problem.[12]

Provide an infirmary for every school district. Working families need a place where they can leave sick children. A great deal of infection is spread because children are sent to school when they should be kept at home, often because there is no one with whom to leave them at home. An infirmary that provides minimal nursing care would fill this vacuum in available medical service.

Locate preventive medical facilities in close proximity to recreational facilities. The identification of health maintenance with pleasurable activities would help overcome some of the resistance to medical examinations.

Provide buses to transport mothers and children to needed health services. A great obstacle to the use of medical services is their inaccessibility. Where and when necessary, buses should be available to bring parents and children to appropriate medical facilities.

Provide mobile units equipped with facilities for diagnosis, treatment, and rehabilitation for use in rural areas where medical services are inaccessible or in urban areas where people are reluctant to leave their immediate locale to seek medical care. This is now a society on wheels. Mobile libraries, homes, and even playgrounds are increasing. The variety of mobile multiphasic and other health units already developed can be extended to guarantee penetration into all areas and to meet an increasing variety of health needs and services.[13]

Furthermore, such mobile units can be seen as part of the larger effort to limit reliance on the polluting private automobile.

## Provide New Institutional Forms

Today the skyrocketing costs for hospitalization, coupled with new forms of medical treatment, make it both feasible and economically essential to treat many aspects of illness away from the hospital, in less intense and less expensive environments.[14] Projected alternatives to hospitalization include programs involving, singly or in combination, day hospitals, night hospitals, convalescent settings, rehabilitative centers, home care, medical foster care, and parent-child hostels for use while a child undergoes diagnostic procedures. These alternate accommodations for children who are currently occupying hospital beds would provide less expensive, more suitable institutional forms for dealing with illness after it has occurred.

### DAY HOSPITALS AND NIGHT HOSPITALS

Hospitalizing a child who does not need around-the-clock medical supervision is expensive and risks unnecessary behavioral upsets owing to separation from family. In many cases, satisfactory medical treatment or diagnosis can be accomplished through the hospitalization of a child for a portion of the day. Certain patients with psychiatric disorders can be successfully treated by involvement in day or night therapeutic inpatient environments, coupled with outside involvement in the home or on the job. The same principle of partial care in specially designed settings is recommended for children who do not need around-the-clock medical supervision, as well as for convalescent or chronically ill patients requiring limited activity. Such day hospitals can be planned to accommodate the need for rest, surveillance, and therapy as well as for school and recreation.[15]

Patients needing therapy requiring mechanical equipment or special treatment for several hours each day can benefit from integrated daytime programs of medical care, school, and recreation. In a night hospital setting a child undergoing dialysis, for example, can spend days with his family at home, sleeping in the hospital when dialysis is necessary. Another form of day hospital provides for minor surgery procedures, which can be performed in the morning so that a child can safely return home at night.[16]

## *Design Guidelines*

Provide day hospitals and night hospitals adjacent to acute medical facilities and integrated with school and recreational programs. Prototypes for these facilities must be developed to explore the most satisfactory locations as well as the most effective ways to group children with different disease patterns and physical requirements.

Provide bus and ambulance services to transport children between the day or night hospitals and their homes. Many programs already provide transportation of physically or mentally handicapped children to special schools. This type of service would be a logical extension of part-time hospital programs as well.

**PEDIATRIC HOME CARE**

Historically, hospital care was reserved for the poor. Those who could afford to paid the physician to make house calls and cared for their sick at home. Today, home care is again advocated for the many pediatric patients who do not require all the specialized staff, equipment, and services of the hospital. "Home care has numerous forms. It varies from programs offering single services such as nursing care of the sick at home, homemaker-home health aid or meals-on-wheels, to multiservice patterns." [17] English physicians who have operated home care programs report that many therapeutic and diagnostic procedures can be carried out successfully in the home.[18] Medical students who have been assigned home care patients have benefited directly from the opportunity to see patients in their own home environments.[19]

Paradoxically, at a time when it is medically possible and economically necessary to reduce the medical services given at the highly specialized acute hospital sites, the condition of poor housing and poverty in people's homes, the reluctance of physicians to make house calls, and the lack of available ambulant services hardly make this choice feasible. In many homes there is neither the space, the time, the food, nor the care available to accommodate the carefully prescribed regimens necessary for convalescence and rehabilitation. Home care, therefore, will not be a realistic alternative for many until high-quality, low-cost housing is more generally available, until parents can get paid sick leave when their children are sick, until the home can be adapted and equipped to meet the needs of the chronically ill and disabled, and until home support programs such as visiting nurse, mobile nursing units, and mobile clinics are adequately supplied.[20]

## *Design Guidelines*

Provide adequate homemaking and medical services to ensure a proper environment for the care of children.

Develop communication links between home and school to keep children in communication with their peer groups.

Link home-care programs with appropriate medical facilities to guarantee high-quality medical supervision of care.

Adapt homes to accommodate to the particular needs of sick and handicapped children easily, to enable them to function at their maximum capacity.

Design house plans flexibly to allow easy substitution of aids to the handicapped, such as ramps instead of steps, grab-bars in bathrooms, wide doorways for wheelchair passage.

MOTELS AND HOSTELS NEAR MEDICAL CENTERS

Today there is an increasing use of regional medical centers for highly complex diagnostic procedures. Patients come from great distances for these services and require adequate accommodations nearby. Both because of inadequate alternative accommodations and because many insurance plans cover only inpatient procedures, acute hospital beds are often used for ambulatory patients undergoing disgnostic procedures. Such practice not only misuses expensive and highly specialized facilities, but also unnecessarily exposes children to the hospital environment.

## *Design Guidelines*

Provide inexpensive motels and hostels near medical centers for children undergoing diagnostic procedures and their families. Work toward acceptance of this expense by health insurance companies and welfare agencies.

Provide recreational facilities for free time and for adult supervision of siblings.

# The Hospital and the Community 2

Despite the growing number of alternative medical care facilities and systems, the need continues to hospitalize some children, on both short- and long-term bases. The treatment of many congenital disorders, metabolic problems, accidents, and surgical conditions requires the specialized environment of the hospital. Types of hospitals will necessarily vary, depending on the types of care given. Some hospitals are geared for acute illness, while others specialize in rehabilitation or longer-term care. A children's hospital differs in various ways from a general hospital with a pediatric unit.

A key planning problem involves the location, size, and type of hospital, relative to specific geographic areas and medical care systems. The alternatives to hospitals, such as facilities for ambulant patients near where people live, work, and go to school, must in turn have some link to the hospital, should a patient require its more specialized services. There are many ways to design a coordinated system for medical service. Such a system can link ambulant facilities like medical clinics, private doctors' offices, or school-based medical facilities to a larger medical clinic or to a hospital. Several hospitals, in turn, can be linked to a university medical center. Maximum utilization of both professional time and high-cost diagnostic and therapeutic equipment can result from centralization of these services. The hospital then becomes only one aspect of a "medical park," which can also accommodate such facilities as a motel for ambulant or convalescent patients, a hostel for visiting relatives or patients undergoing diagnostic tests, and a convalescent home. A separate ambulant facility can also be included on the same site. The pattern of care and the linkage between the component parts are affected by the geography of the area, the existing medical facilities, and the demographic nature of the population and their medical needs. The parts of the system can be linked either by a close physical proximity or by jitney service and computers. It is essential to locate the facility so that it can be easily used by the group it serves and so that there is an accepted and understood pattern of use. The community must know where to go for emergency, acute, or routine care.

Some of the new facilities and staffing patterns recommended here may cost additional money, but these changes are in some cases as vital to recovery as any other medical treatment component. Other of the recommendations, however, can be accomplished without additional cost. In any case, it is false economy to cure a child of a physical ailment only to induce a psychological one. In terms of national priorities, it would seem that moneys should be allocated to cure children right here in this country rather than to destroy other children elsewhere.

## Allow Decision-Making by Users

Perhaps the single most important factor affecting the social, emotional, and developmental needs of children in a hospital setting is the attitude of parents and staff toward each other. Hostility, fear, and mistrust among the medical personnel, administration, and parents prevent the development of a treatment environment sympathetic to the child's needs. In order to feel comfortable and at ease, a child and his parents need the reassurance and comfort of staff who speak their language and understand their home conditions and patterns of life.

Today an atmosphere of mistrust separates some persons who come from low socioeconomic backgrounds and who inhabit the ghettos of the cities from the so-called medical establishment. This mistrust is based partly on years of unpleasant hospital experience, which has created an image of the hospital as alien. If this is to be overcome and mutual trust is to be created, the community must participate in the decision processes of the hospital in terms of both its internal and external policy.[1]

The need to bridge the gap between the medical consumer, particularly the low-income consumer, and the hospital has long been recognized.[2] The introduction of community workers representing diverse ethnic and economic groups has begun to play a role in improving patient-hospital staff relations. Attempts are also being made to obtain opinions from diverse groups in the community. Ultimately, full community involvement at all levels of decision-making is essential.[3]

Meaningful architectural guidelines can be developed only from a shared understanding of health goals and the means of achieving them among all users, whether doctor, patient, administrator, or nurse. The process of developing a shared image is an educational process, which occurs over time. It is not enough to ask users what they want; one must also equip them with the knowledge of possible alternatives and consequences.

### *Design Guidelines*

Include all categories of consumers as well as health professionals, administrators, and employees on all decision-making bodies. As with any interdisciplinary group learning to work together, these mixed decision-making bodies will have to overcome major communications barriers, but it should be possible, in an atmosphere of mutual trust, to sort out general spheres of concern. For example, consumers will have minimal interest or expertise in surgical theater design or policy and maximal interest in setting social patterns on the nursing unit.

Provide instruction for health workers and members of the community in understanding physical plans, including a wide variety of visual aids in both two and three dimensions, as well as visits to existing facilities to relate constructed forms to scale drawings. In many cases the user, whether an administrator, doctor, or community member, will otherwise misread the plans and, assuming he is to get one thing, will be surprised when the building is completed and he receives quite another.

## Design for Accessibility, Reassurance, and Human Scale

The design of a hospital is a complex matter. Natural conditions of site and climate modify design, as do technical constraints of structure, mechanical systems, methods of communication, legal restrictions, and available money. Together these factors help determine the form of a pediatric facility. Yet pressure to fulfill these many requirements must not lead one to ignore the image that the hospital presents to the community — an image that will affect community use of the facility.

Even before a child enters the hospital, he has an image of it. If the hospital looks like a fortress, he can imagine being locked up there, and he reacts with fear. This kind of impression represents a major problem of modern institutions. They have grown in scale to such a size that their physical expression is monumental rather than human. This tendency has been encouraged both by the notion that efficiency and size are synonymous and by the feeling of satisfaction derived by administrators and donors from large-scale projects.

Similarly, largeness has resulted in creating an attitude of irresponsibility on the part of users. Hard, shiny materials are chosen instead of materials that mellow with age and generate an atmosphere of warmth. The building tells the user that he need not become involved.

In contrast, attempts to improve the hospital may lead to designing a facility that is "too nice" for some patients. The hospital environment may be so much better than his home environment that a child may wish not to leave. Dr. Donald Fink, a pediatric psychiatrist, notes that when a child wishes to stay in the hospital, his service takes this as an important signal that both the child and his home may need help from the community.[4]

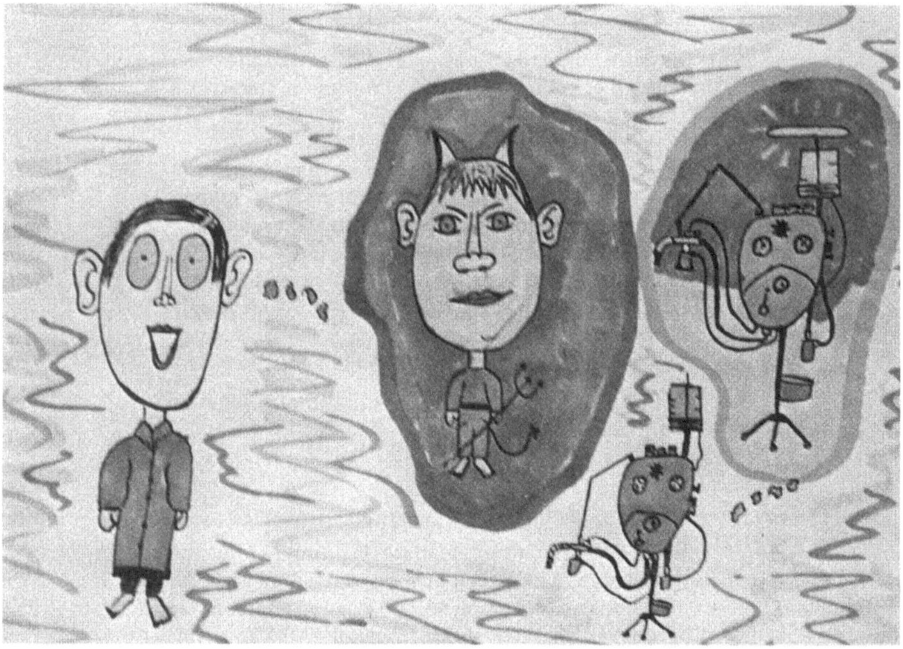

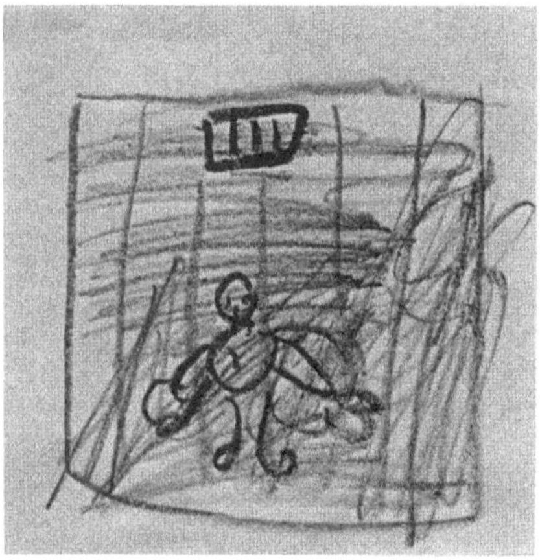

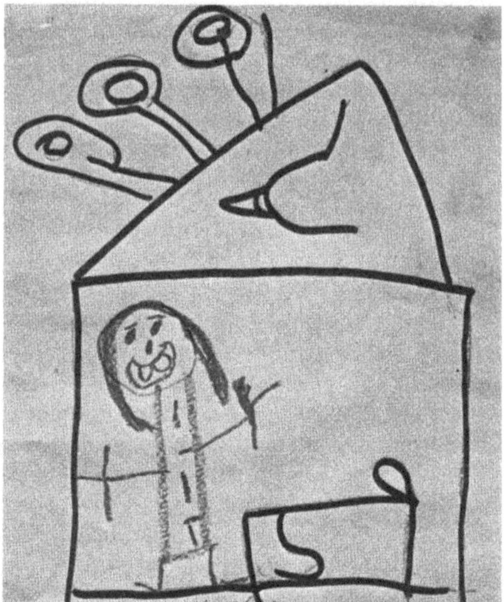
(Girl in hospital)

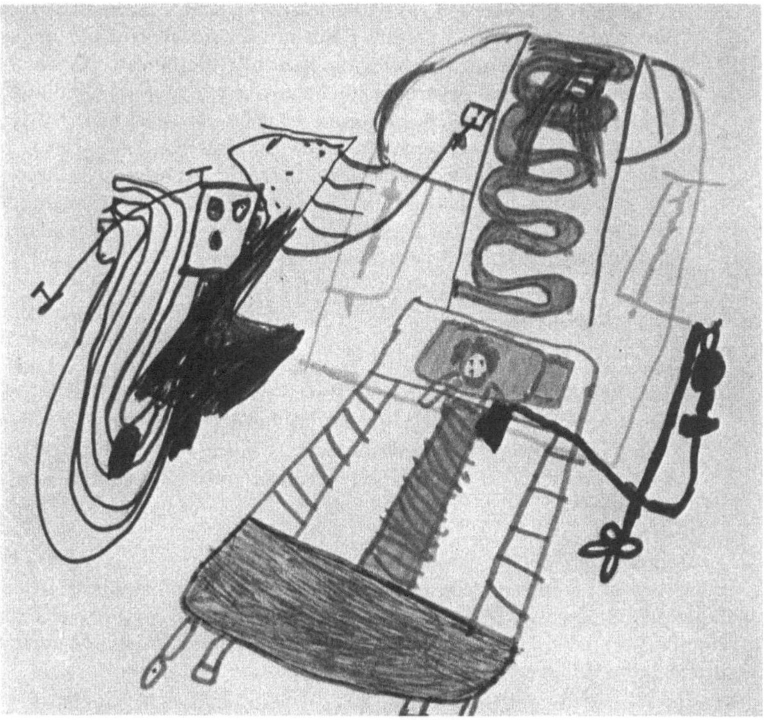

ENTRY TO THE HOSPITAL

Before entering the hospital, many children will have had some form of preparation. Excellent books have been written for various age groups explaining hospital routines visually and in terms that children can understand. Some school children visit hospitals after studying these books and see for themselves the peculiarities of hospital routine. If later they must be hospitalized, some of the unfamiliarity and scariness of hospitalization has been removed.

Even if the hospital presents a pleasant and welcoming image to the community, entry into the hospital on short notice through the emergency unit can negatively affect the whole hospital experience. From the moment a child catches his first sight of the hospital, his eyes are wide open, watchful for dangers and anxious to keep track of where he is and who is responsible for him. Lucy Muldrow, a nurse and mother, describes a typical emergency experience:

> A child breaks a bone while playing at school. He lands in a hospital via ambulance — several anxious teachers around — near panic because of the difficulty in immediately reaching his parent.

> His parent is contacted on the job or at home, pushes the panic button, races to the Emergency Room, and finds his child covered with blood. He is not aware of the extent of the illness. Nurses and doctors rush around — sick people lie all around, moaning and groaning. The child is already in a state of shock because of the injury, not to mention the anxiety shown on the parent's face. The nurse and doctor by this time have made the child as comfortable as possible and attempted to reassure the family with their limited time. They try to console other families or care for someone in more danger of dying than the child with the broken bone.
>
> In the meantime, the child is carted off to the X-ray department. Parents may or may not accompany the child. Depending on institution — the child may be left in the hall strapped to the gurney, because a man with head injuries from an auto accident needs attention first. The child may or may not be screened and possibly will see the man with all the bandages on his head and hear him groaning with pain. Finally he is wheeled into the X-ray room for the picture-taking process — those gigantic machines probably remind him of monsters.[5]

Whether approaching through the emergency entrance or otherwise, another aspect of entering the hospital that alienates the family is the red tape and bureaucracy associated with admission. Often a variety of forms for the hospital and insurance or welfare plans must be signed prior to making the child comfortable.

## *Design Guidelines*

Make the child's path pleasant, simple, and direct between family car, taxi, bus, or ambulance and nursing unit.

Provide a separate entrance for pediatric patients, as well as a separate emergency entrance and waiting area.

Connect the pediatric emergency area to the nursing unit by a special elevator or short corridor.

Assign personnel to individual patients so that the same registered or licensed vocational nurse who admits a patient takes him to x-ray, cares for him on the unit, and tends to many of his other needs.

Delay completing entry procedures until after the child has been made comfortable in his hospital unit.

CIRCULATION AND WAITING

Once inside the hospital, the child and his family may feel dwarfed by its huge size and depressed by the concentration of human suffering. Hospital circulation patterns are generally so complex, involving several changes of level and direction, that adults as well as children feel lost.[6] Trips from the nursing unit to other hospital sections through hallways cluttered with strange equipment or lined with alarmingly ill patients can intensify the anxiety of a child headed for a new and possibly painful experience. Efforts must be made to make linkages as direct, short, and pleasant as possible.

Once at the point of destination, children and parents may spend tedious minutes or hours waiting to be examined, tested, and treated. Much of this tiring, wasteful waiting could be avoided through closer scheduling. Yet because trained medical personnel are in short supply and medical practice is unpredictable, some waiting is inevitable. Waiting time can and should be used productively.

## *Design Guidelines*

Avoid the labyrinthine paths so common in very large buildings.

Make corridors pleasant by using warm colors and surfaces, by carpeting the floor, by using diffused lighting, by locating stops of interest along the way, and by opening the perspective at intervals to interesting views.

Locate other nursing units and services off the main corridors so that it is never necessary to pass through them on the way from the pediatric nursing unit to any other service.

Provide generous storage off the corridor so that equipment need not be stored in constant view.

Provide waiting areas for the sicker patients off the corridor and include interesting things for children to do, such as toys, paper and crayons, books, and quiet games. In many areas educational displays can be used. For example, an x-ray department waiting room might have posters showing how the machines work and supply discarded plates for children to examine. Most displays should be interesting to parents as well as children. To be engrossing, displays need not take health as a theme. Many other topics presented in sufficiently vivid detail can be diverting and educational.

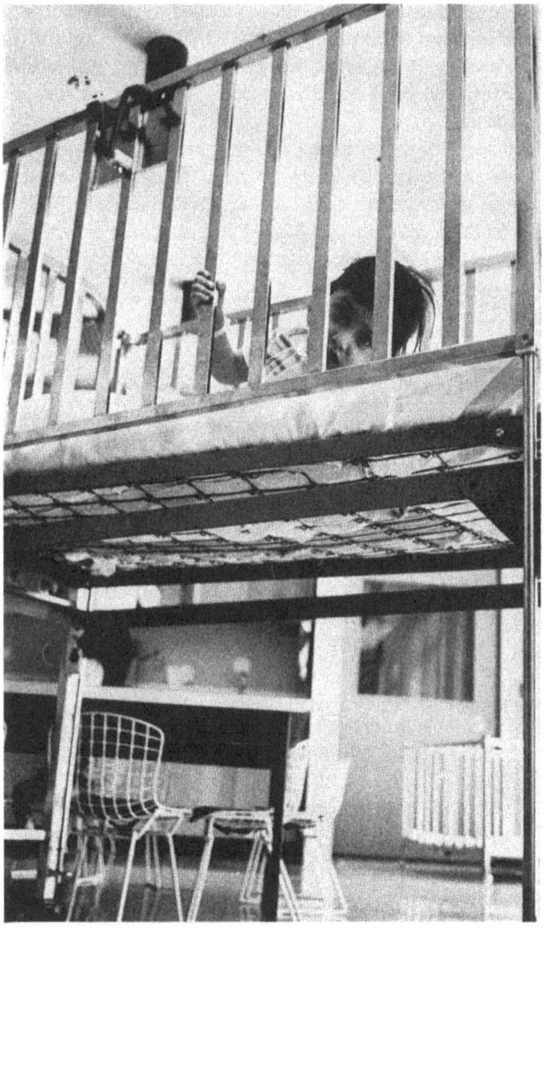

# Infants 3

An infant (0–12 months) has basic needs for physical care. If he is not fed and kept clean, warm, and safe, he will die. His own early attachment to his mother — made up of such responses as sucking, clinging, following, crying, and smiling — helps to assure his survival.[1] Less is known about his other needs, but increasing evidence shows that an infant needs to be held, cuddled, talked to, cooed at, and visually and tactually stimulated, or his developmental progress will be adversely affected.[2] According to Peter Wolf and Richard Feinbloom, who find social and cognitive development to be functionally inseparable, social attachment in early life is prerequisite to later learning.[3]

Catherine Landreth writes: "Vocalizing to a baby and responding to his vocalizations will make him more vocal. Smiling, communicating with him in motor play, and responding to his social overtures will make him more socially responsive and outgoing. Giving him an opportunity to practice his emerging sensory-motor skills will help him find out what he can do and what his world is like."[4] Reporting on animal studies involving various species of infant mammals, Wolf and Feinbloom conclude that immature visual and motor systems require stimulation in order to maintain and develop structure.

Thus, optimum environments for infants provide early opportunities for the stimulation and development of social responsiveness, language and motor skills, and the cognitive function. Further, the early relationships of infants with supportive and responsive adults enhance their capacities to form mature relationships in later life.

Much of the evidence showing the effect of maladaptive early infant environments on later behavioral characteristics was derived from studies of children in institutions. These institutions generally were poor, overcrowded, and understaffed. The children, seldom cuddled or picked up, had few toys. Even enlightened institutions placed emphasis on cleanliness and adequate food rather than on personal contact, cuddling, and vocalization.[5] The environments for such infants shared many similar characteristics — isolating the children and depriving them of contact with family and each other, as well as with things to see and to do. When maintained for weeks or months in such settings, infants showed severe effects.[6] The term "hospitalism" refers to gross developmental retardation and personality distortion seen in infants institutionalized and maternally deprived during the first year. It was coined by René Spitz, who showed that early separation affects later social development most profoundly when it takes place during the first two years of life.[7] Infants experiencing severe deprivation through prolonged institutionalization showed long-lasting, sometimes seemingly irreversible, impairment in intellectual and social functioning, language and motor development.[8] In contrast, other experimental studies have shown that planned intensive mothering of infants, even in an institutional setting, can result in increased social responsiveness and vocalization.[9]

Studies on the reaction of sick infants to hospitalization demonstrate many of the same responses seen in institutionalized children, depending on the type of sickness, the duration of the experience, and the age at which it occurs.[10] The very young infant generally experiences no ill effects from hospitalization and the separation from his mother or the familiar person caring for him as long as his needs for food, warmth, and love are met by an adequate "mother substitute." According to John Bowlby, the infant only gradually develops the ability to respond differentially to a familiar mother figure and the stranger, but by six months "he comes to center his instinctual responses not only on a human figure but on a particular human figure." [11]

These observations are consistent with those of H. R. Schaffer and W. M. Callender, who studied the reactions of infants under one year of age to short-term hospitalization.[12] In the hospital, babies under seven months showed little protest at separation from their mothers, easily accepted a stranger as mother substitute, and adjusted well to changed feeding routines. The older infants, between seven and twelve months, showed a markedly different pattern — initial protest, negativism toward staff, and subdued, withdrawn behavior. The longer-term effects of the hospital experience were less noticeable in the younger infants, who nonetheless showed decreased vocalization, increased proccupation with the environment, and short-lived sleep and feeding disturbances. The older infants showed more severe reactions: extreme dependence on their mothers, anxiety about separation and strangers, and sleep disturbances.

## Minimize Number of Persons Caring for Infant

If a parent cannot be present in the hospital, the hospital should first try to determine why and to provide the necessary services to enable the parent to be present with his sick child, and next it should organize the work so that "nurses can be assigned to particular children to care for them in all ways, so that each child may feel he has a secure relationship with one real person." [13] In general, both in hospitals and in child care centers for infants, one adult can care for three to five infants if they do not require intensive nursing. In Soviet nurseries, each "upbringer" has responsibility for four infants.[14] In a kibbutz infants house, one adult and two full-time assistants can take care of a maximum of sixteen infants ranging in age from four days to one year.[15] At Stanford University Medical Center, Stanford, California, a full-time nurse cares for four infants with occasional help from other pediatric nurses. In proposing ways to reduce problems resulting from "multiple mothering" and thus to improve residential care for infants, Louise Sandler and Barbara Topic suggest that "family" structures in nurseries contain no more than three infants per "mother," as part of a maximum family of ten children.[16]

Many hospitals combine infants with toddlers and preschoolers in one nursing unit. Points of view differ as to the advantages and disadvantages of this grouping arrangement. The advantages lie chiefly in the additional attention and stimulation afforded to the infants by the presence of slightly older children who can both talk to them and provide them with interesting activity to watch. Some older children in turn benefit from the experience of helping with the babies. On the negative side of the ledger, staff members sometimes prefer working with infants rather than toddlers, or vice versa, and are most skilled at handling the age group they prefer. Nurses claim more staffing is necessary if infants are to be mixed with toddlers and preschoolers.[17] The different sleeping and eating habits and the difference in capabilities require constant supervision lest, with the best intentions in the world, an older child injure a younger one.

## *Design Guidelines*

Provide one adult staff member for every three to five infants.

Provide a small, self-contained subunit for each three, four, or five infants within a larger nursing unit accommodating all children under six. There should be visual control of all persons entering and leaving the subunit.

Provide movable screens for darkening individual crib areas for napping. This is essential where age groups are to be mixed.

Enable the nurse to administer total care to the children in an infant subunit of four cribs by providing complete facilities for crawling, bathing, rocking, and feeding.

Provide garbage and laundry chutes or other means of collecting waste and dirty linen from the outside.

Locate an examination and treatment space and nurses' toilet near and accessible to the crib room.

## Allow Maximum Contact with Parent or Nurse

The infant first derives his contact and image of the outside world from his response to feeding and its associated pleasurable sensations. This is generally a time when the mother or mother substitute rocks and sings to the infant and cuddles him.[18] In addition to the satisfaction from relieving hunger, the infant gets warmth, sensory contact, and rhythmic and auditory experience.[19] The continuation of warm bodily contact and a rhythmic and auditory experience in the hospital is especially important since the infant cannot understand where he is or why he is there, and depends for support on familiar activities, even if the people are unfamiliar.

### *Design Guidelines*

Provide alcoves with rocking chairs for parents or nurses to feed the infants. A feeding alcove should accommodate two adults.

Provide the possibility of privacy in the alcove if a nursing mother so desires.

Provide maximum opportunities for parent participation, including live-in accommodations, particularly if the child is over six months.

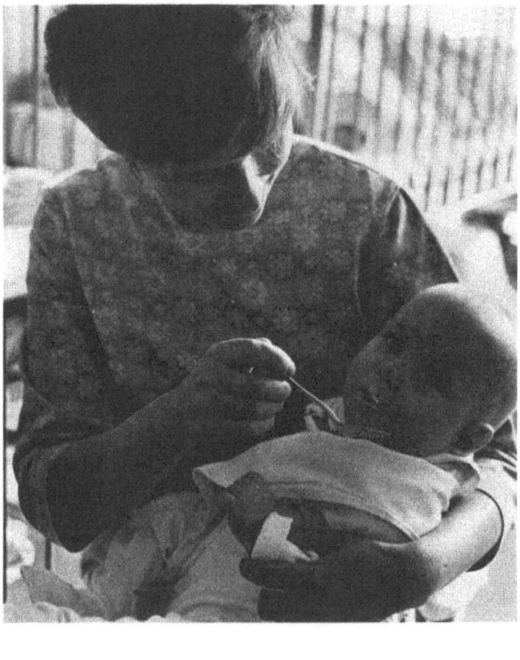

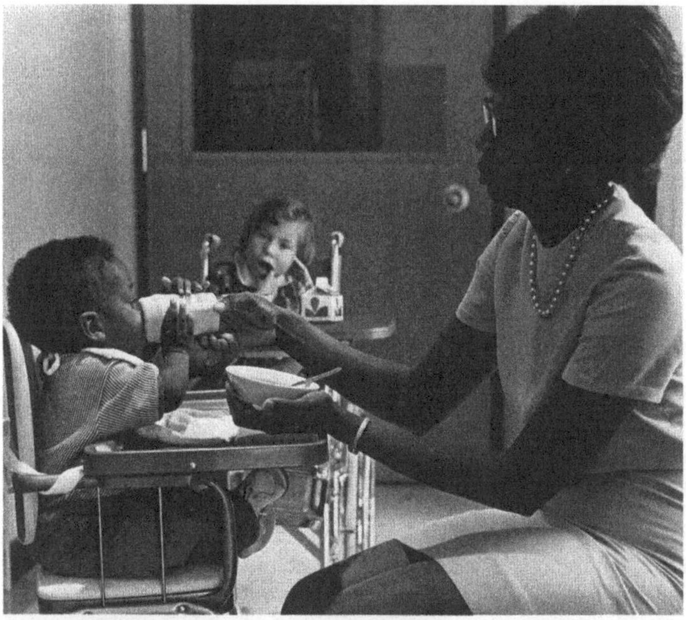

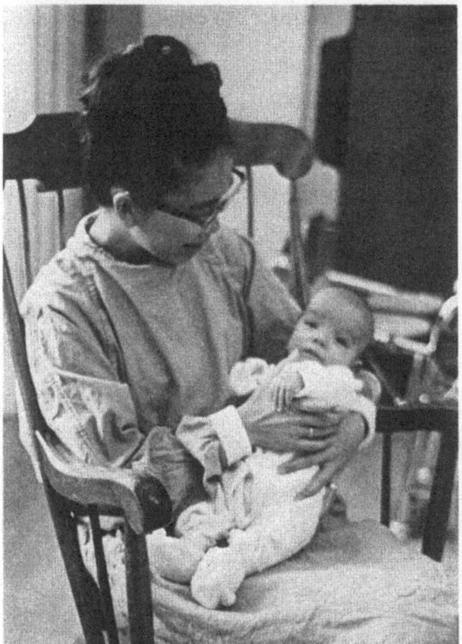

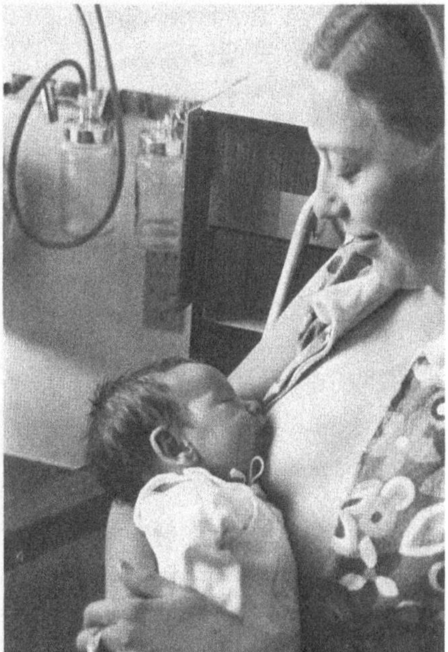

## Provide Places To Develop Motor Skills

In the first year of life an infant learns to creep and crawl, to stand up, and finally to take a few steps. Opportunities must be provided for the infant to exercise his new-found skills. Infants in hospitals are often confined to cribs because there is no safe area in which to play and learn. In the standard hospital crib room, a variety of wheeled goods, sharp corners, light plugs, oxygen tanks, and other equipment make an infant's exploration on the floor perilous. A nurse who is responsible for several infants can seldom take the time away from other duties to give a crawling infant the constant supervision needed.

The standard home playpen is used in some hospitals, but it offers the infant little more than the crib. In such a small place his creeping and crawling are restricted. In attempting to counteract the feeling of deep loss experienced by infants separated from their mothers through hospitalization, Emma Plank found that "a change in environment away from the crib is stimulating in itself and encourages babies to move. They enjoy playing on a mat, moving in a walker, or being in a rocker or a baby swing." [20]

In the Soviet Union, "infants are placed in group playpens with six to eight children in each. To permit face-to-face interaction between staff members and children the pens are raised on legs, the one for the three-to-six-month olds being higher than that for the near toddlers." [21] The raised location, in addition to allowing the infant more familiarity with his nurse's face than with her shoes, has the obvious advantage of limiting the stooping and lifting necessary when children are on the floor.

### *Design Guidelines*

Provide a "giant playpen" or small enclosed alcove off a larger space for crawling infants, in full view of the nursing substation.

Provide a large space with sturdy tables for infants to pull themselves up and walk around, boxes to sit in, and toys as required.

Provide a warm, soft floor.

Eliminate electrical outlets, wheeled goods, and other hazards from this crawling area.

Provide outdoor crawling areas with a soft surface (grass or outdoor carpet), fully supervizable from nursing substation.

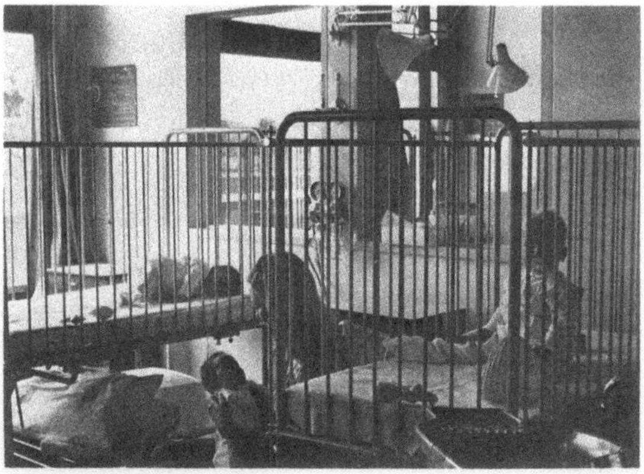

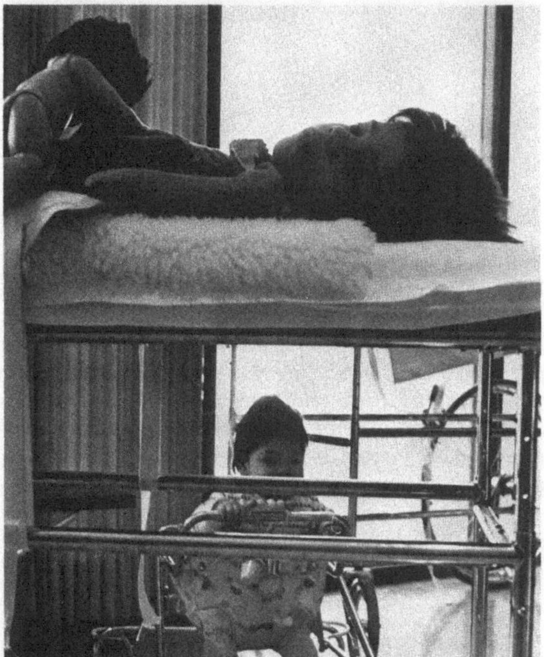

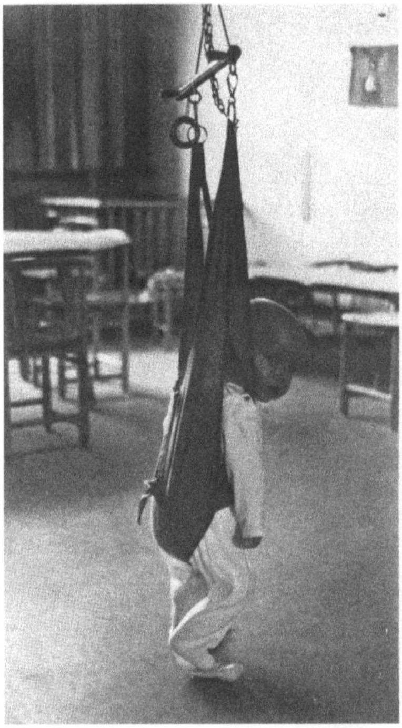

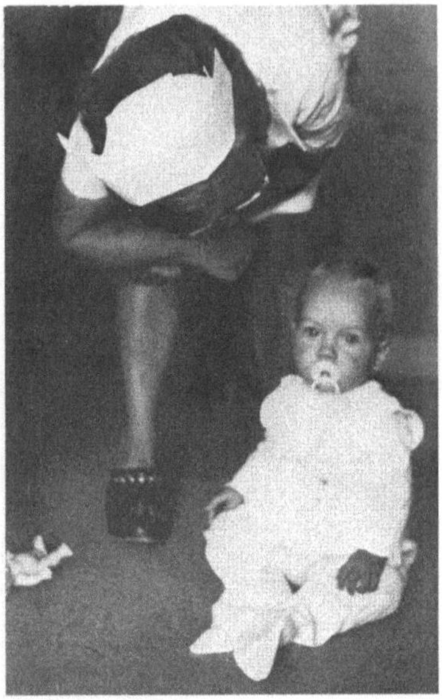

## Provide Stimulating Sensory Experiences

Sensory stimulation of many kinds is now recognized as a necessary environmental condition for infant development. Touching and playing with water and food, crawling on diverse floor textures, playing with a variety of toys, watching the changes of light and shadow as the sun moves across a room — all add stimulation to the environment. Millar has described the infant's response to sensory stimuli as follows:

> When babies are awake and comfortable, they spend their time looking, listening, and generally responding in a way which has led people to describe them as "hungry" for stimuli. This becomes more obvious as they grow older. A five-month-old may find it difficult to go on eating if anything else interesting is going on, and I have known a hungry one-year-old refuse his bottle with screams of indignation because it obscured his view of the pretty pattern on his new pyjamas.
> The common practice of hanging rattles on babies' cots probably originated as magic to frighten off evil spirits. But brightly coloured rattles hung where the baby can see them, and hear the noise they make, do avert boredom. Swaying branches, pictures and patterned curtains are stared at with unblinking intensity by young infants.[22]

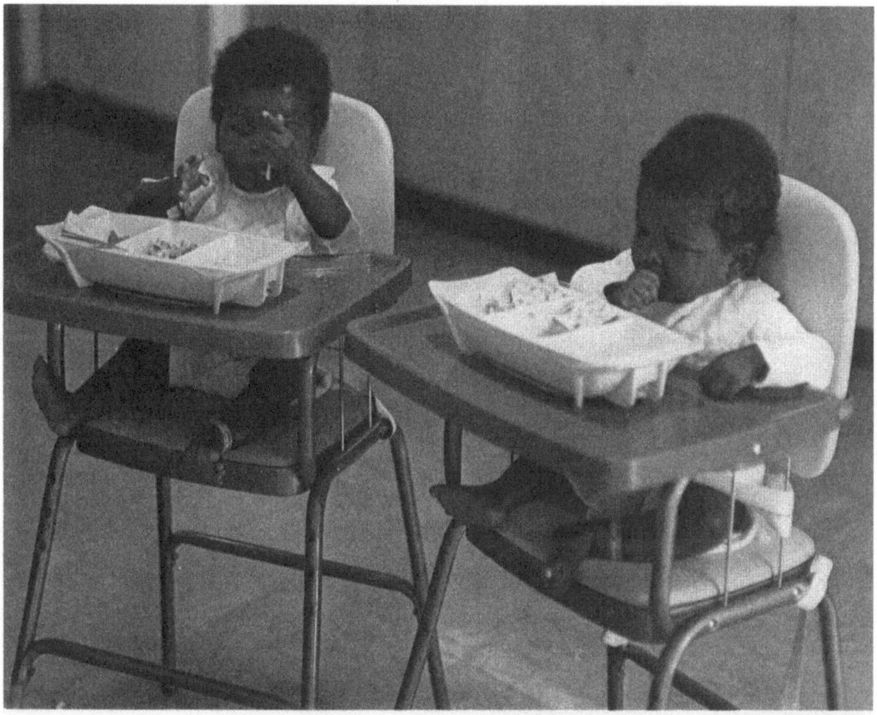

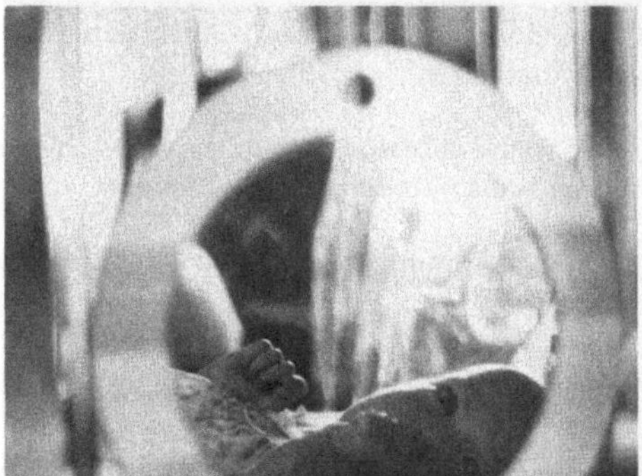

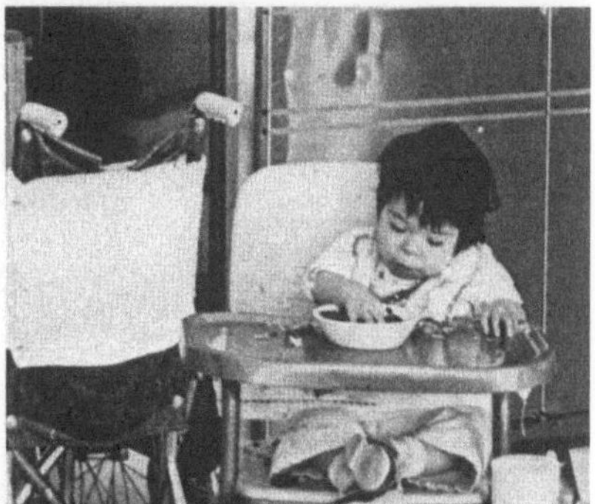

Hospital architects have assumed that infants do not require the visual, tactile, and auditory stimulus required by older children and adults. Too many infant facilities still exist that include rows of white cots in interior rooms with absolutely no relief from the starkness and monotony. Experimental psychologists who were exploring the perceptual interests of infants noted: "Some babies, from the age of two weeks onwards, began to show signs of boredom at being repeatedly shown a moving metal disc. They started looking away at the white surroundings, then repeatedly had a sneaking look at the object, apparently having some sort of game." [23] To remedy this situation, designers painted white walls in pastel colors, then in bright colors with intense patches of pure blue, red, and orange. Actually, experiments indicate that infants prefer patterns to colors, and complex patterns like bull's eyes and black-and-white checkerboards to simple forms like triangles and squares. In one such experiment, six different disks were shown to infants: a face, a piece of printed matter, a bull's eye, and plain red, white, and yellow disks. Even the youngest infants preferred patterns over color.[24]

## *Design Guidelines*

Provide a sunny and light atmosphere. Natural lighting is essential.

Use textured materials near the infants. Mobiles with different tactile properties should hang within reach.

Use patterned materials. Patterned mobiles should hang from the ceiling. Patterned curtains should cover the windows. Staff should be allowed to select colorful patterned and textured clothing.

Allow infants to watch different types of activity — nurses at work, children at play, trees outside the window.

Use music, as well as stimulating the infants by talking to them.

# Toddlers and Preschoolers 4

Between the age at which a child first walks and the age he enters school, he grows and develops more than during any other five-year period in his life. At one, most children can stand alone and are learning to walk, though a one-year-old will still resort to crawling for real speed. By three a child has begun to master his body. He can balance on one foot, jump, and pedal a tricycle. Between three and six, a child further advances in physical strength, coordination, and manual dexterity. He can run, jump, climb, roll, tumble and somersault.

Learning to talk is another developmental milestone. At one, a child communicates his basic needs through sounds and motions. He knows several words that may be used to fill many needs. "Ma-ma" may be an all-purpose vocalization, signaling the child's desire for food, a clean diaper, comfort, or sleep. The rate of development of language skills is especially variable: some three-year-olds talk extensively; others use only a few words to communicate. In bilingual households toddlers will often communicate in a mixture of the two languages, understandable only to parents and bilingual personnel. Between three and six a child's understanding and use of words develop to include the ability to define many common objects. He begins to express some of his feelings verbally.

These age differentials are by no means rigid. As a child develops from a clumsy toddler to a coordinated six-year-old, he follows a highly individual pattern of development. One child will play cooperatively with others at twenty months, another not until three-and-one-half years. Coordination, vocabulary, social relations, and self-help capability in toileting, dressing, eating, and washing vary with each child.

Hospitalization is a threat to most young children. A toddler left in the hospital feels betrayed and deserted. He is too young to understand assurances that his parents will return and that he will soon go home. A three-year-old in the hospital may understand a little more — when his parents leave, for example, he can usually understand their promise to return — but no words can overcome his fear of being left alone nor the

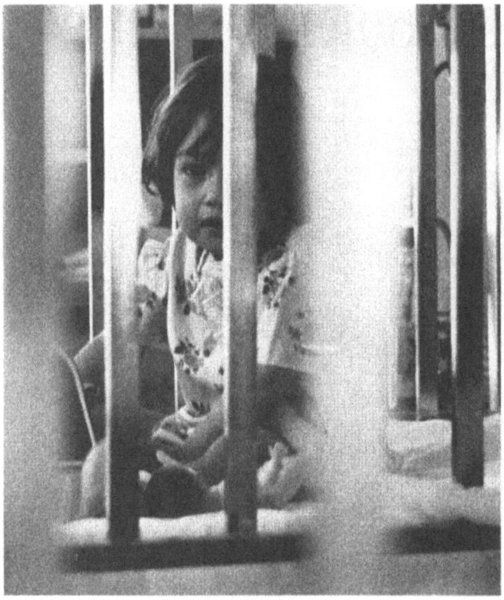

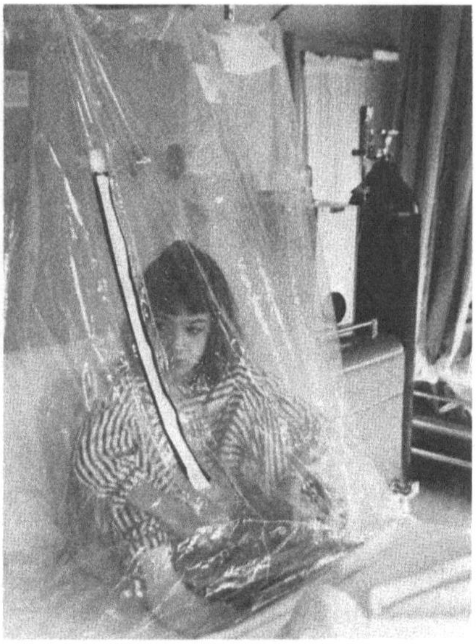

tension he feels at the sight of hospital equipment. His lack of time sense further accentuates his feeling of abandonment.

The older preschool child can understand more of what hospitalization means, especially if it has been carefully explained to him, but his newly developed fears of bodily harm or mutilation interfere with his adjustment to the hospital.[1] The sight of oxygen tents and of the nylon netting or plastic domes sometimes put over a crib to keep agile preschoolers from escaping only reinforces his feelings of being trapped and defenseless. One play therapist interviewed by the authors reported that when she had been placed in an oxygen tent as a child, she had thought the hospital staff was trying to kill her, because her mother had warned her strongly against playing with plastic bags.

Toddlers often respond to hospitalization with a developmental regression to excessive nighttime fears, increased clinging to and dependence on parents, loss of bowel and bladder control, or intensified thumbsucking. The older preschooler may manifest regressive behavior typical of a much younger child. Reversal to bedwetting at this age is not uncommon, nor are increased masturbation, nightmares at night, and disturbances in the relation with parents.[2]

Many doctors now advocate that, if at all possible, the parents stay in the hospital with the child under five. Physicians try to avoid voluntary hospitalization and elective operations on children from three to six because of the child's deep fears of bodily injury.

Much has been written of the traumatic experience of hospitalization.

Yet not only can some of the trauma be mitigated, but the hospital experience itself can be turned into a positive experience in which the child is given opportunities to develop and learn. The child's negative reaction to the hospital experience is in part owing to the fact that the experience is in fact negative. To the end of remedying this situation, the environment for the toddler and preschooler must not only be safe, efficient, and easily supervised, but it must also promote self-help and autonomy in a rich and varied environment that is challenging to the young child relative to his state of development and condition of health.

## Allow for Adequate Visual Supervision at All Times

Hospitalized toddlers and preschool children should be in view of their nurse at all times. They cannot be counted on to use electronic forms of communication. One very worried seven-year-old with a knee infection, who was observed in a hospital by the authors, continually called to the nurse when she was not in view. When the observer got up to leave, he said, "Don't you leave, too!" Even though the child always called to the nurse and never used the available buzzer system, he was able to explain the buzzer system in detail to his visiting grandfather.

Another example of the difficulties experienced by a child with concepts of electronic communication appeared in the press. "The nurse at the desk tried several times to communicate with four-year-old Johnny via the intercom over his bed. At last she said in some exasperation: 'Come on, Johnny, answer me — I know you're there.' After a slight pause, a very frightened little voice asked: 'W-w-what do you want, wall?' "[3]

Because of the difficulty of maintaining continuous, close visual supervision, children in many hospitals are confined to their beds and cribs for long periods during the day, to their detriment. In one community hospital observed, children were confined to their beds and cribs all day, unless a parent was present to take them to the play area. Yet, the thought of the crib as a safe place is an illusion.

In the nursery school environment, adequate supervision of youngsters of preschool age has been defined as the teacher's ability to see whatever is going on in the entire play area merely by taking a few steps. If this criterion were applied to pediatric unit design, very few places would conform. Until recently only the old-fashioned multibed ward configurations have conformed to this standard.

### *Design Guidelines*

Develop the nursing units into a series of substations, each station having all the materials necessary to care effectively for the children in it.

Design a unit as a cluster, with the nurses in the center and the patients' rooms on the periphery. The stations should be organized so that all rooms around a station are immediately visible.[4] This type of organization is used for cardiac and intensive care units, where complete visual monitoring is essential.

If an old unit is being remodeled and a more direct system is not possible, develop a closed circuit television system that allows the nurse to observe the children in each room at all times. The drawback to this system lies in the inability of the child also to see the adult.

Glaze all partitions so that it is possible to see into each room.

Avoid corners and small hallways that obstruct the visual field.

Design the nursing unit with only one, well-controlled entrance. Having several entrances can even lead to molesting, kidnaping, and other avoidable hazards.

## Exclude Equipment Apt To Cause Accidents

Young children are frequently the victims of accidents in the home — more frequently than any other age group. The lack of motor coordination, the slow reaction time, and the lack of experience and hence of judgment typical of a young child make it essential to eliminate as many hazards from his environment as possible.

Once in the hospital, the young child continues to be at a serious risk from accidents. In fact, hospitals have been shown to experience a higher frequency of accidents than do most industries in this country. Most accidents to hospitalized children are caused by falls from either the crib or bed to the floor, or against the side of the bed, as they attempt to climb over the side of the crib or when they lose balance while standing up in bed. In many cases these accidents directly result from the child being unused to a high bed or crib. The second most common cause of accidents is medication errors.[5]

A list of additional hazards and accidents could grow to book size were it to include everything that might lead to injury. It is during this early period of childhood that careful parents empty the lower half of the kitchen cupboard of items that are either sharp, breakable, or poisonous. Obvious danger points particular to the hospital environment must also be watched.[6] At the University of Michigan, Ann Arbor, for example, the Children's Hospital uses only electric beds for children over two. The accident rate has been reduced, and younger children are happier not to revert to a crib.

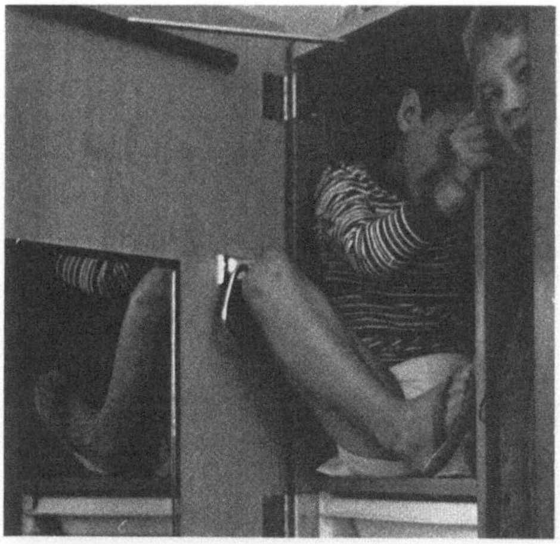

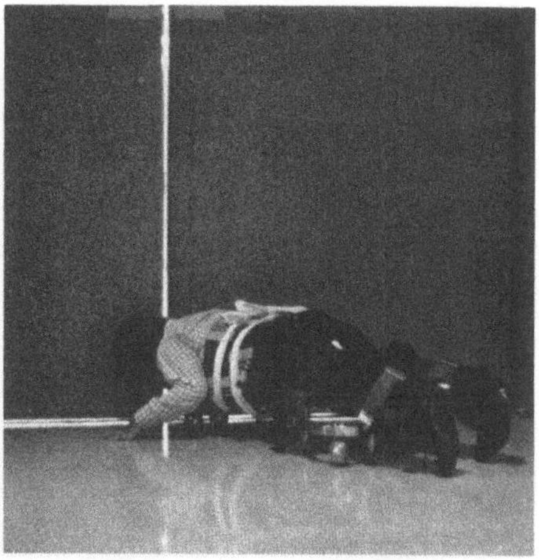

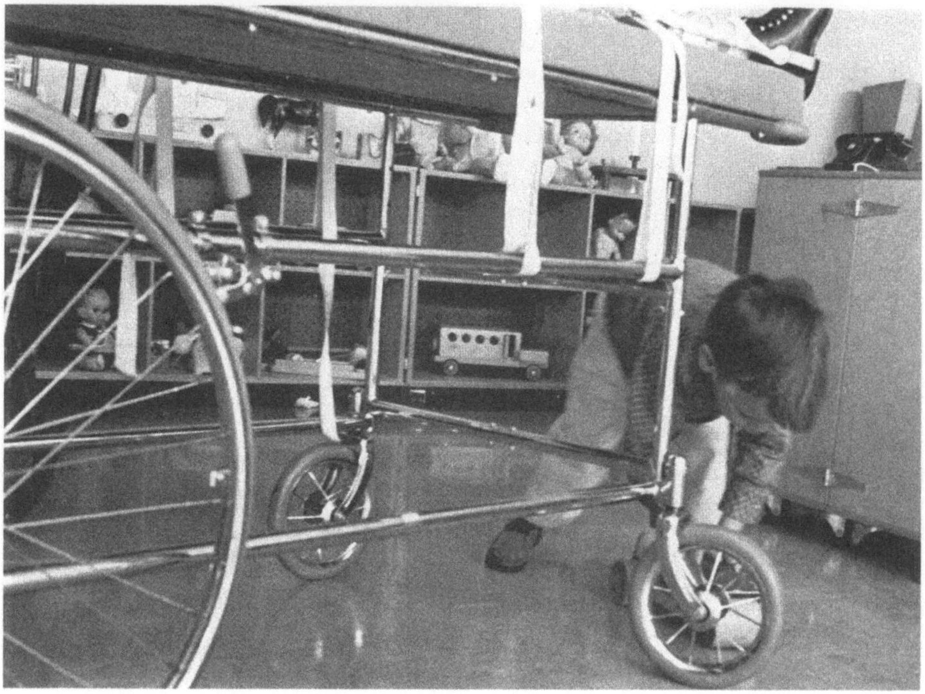

### *Design Guidelines*

Locate oxygen outlets, heaters, electrical outlets, and other potentially dangerous objects out of the reach of children, or at least fifty-five inches high.

Avoid building corners, protruding shelves, or pointed objects in the lower four feet of the room.

Glaze doors at child height to minimize the safety hazard of opening a blind door and hitting an unseen child on the other side.

Use only tempered glass or unbreakable plastic in areas used by children.

Eliminate changes in floor level, as they are hazardous for gurneys, wheelchairs, and crutches. Provide handrails as well.

Provide an isolated area for the preparation of medications, with its own lockable door, sufficiently large for two persons. Provide adequate and carefully marked facilities to store each patient's medications.

Provide electrically controlled cribs, youth beds, or beds that can be raised for the nurse's convenience and lowered to prevent the accidents caused by a youngster's attempts to climb out.

## Maintain Links with Home

Children whose parents cannot be with them in the hospital need to be reassured that they have not been forgotten. There are a number of ways to reassure toddlers and preschoolers. The phone is a source of comfort even to the youngest child, as are tapes of the family, photographs, and movies. Also comforting is a special place for a parent to leave a sweater, glove, or any other familiar possession as a guarantee of his return.

Windows overlooking cars, buses, and parking lots where young patients may see parents arrive and leave provide links to the outer world and give assurance to the young and vulnerable. A teenager has reported that one of her most vivid memories of hospitalization at age four was watching her mother come and go from her window overlooking the hospital parking lot.

*Design Guidelines*



Provide communication equipment such as a telephone, tape recorder, and other means of communicating with home.

Locate windows overlooking the "way home" with sills low enough for the toddler to see over.

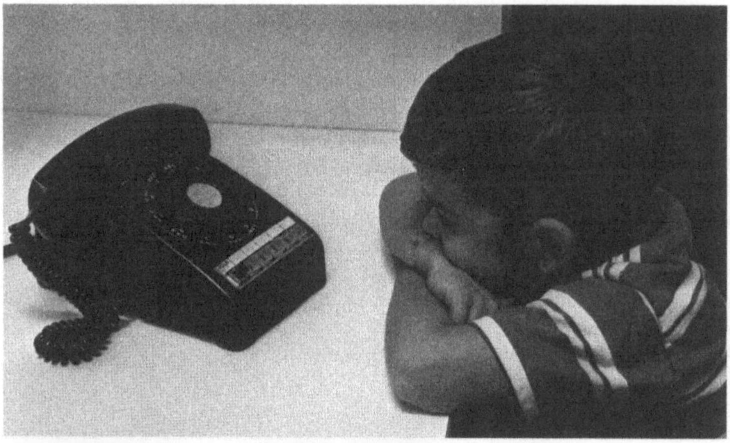

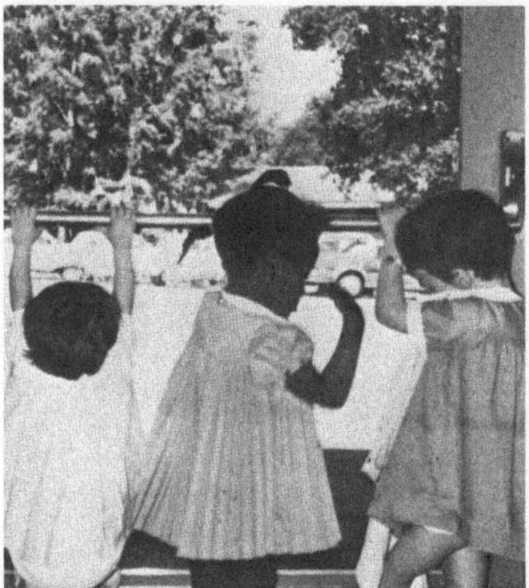

## Accommodate Both Child and Adult Scale

It is customary to think of adapting the environment to the child's scale by altering a few critical dimensions, such as lowering window sill heights and the distance of the bed off the floor.[7] The premise is sound, but to this list must be added certain other dimensions that should also relate to the scale of the child: the heights of sinks and toilets, of cupboards for clothing, of various items such as chairs and tables for eating, of mirrors, and of drinking fountains. Special attention should also be given to the design of the floor, making it free from drafts, warm, soft-surfaced, and adequately lighted.

Doing much more to orient dimensions to child scale, however, would make the environment unworkable for adults. Because of the amount of bending necessarily involved when adults work in a physical environment adapted for young children, such work is physically very demanding, particularly for the nurse who has to render medical treatment in addition to bathing, feeding, playing, and changing.

Perhaps more important than the physical is the social scale of the young child's environment: the size of the peer groups to which the child must relate and the number of adults he encounters. Since children feel most comfortable in small groups, modules of peers should not be larger than twelve, ideally six to eight.[8]

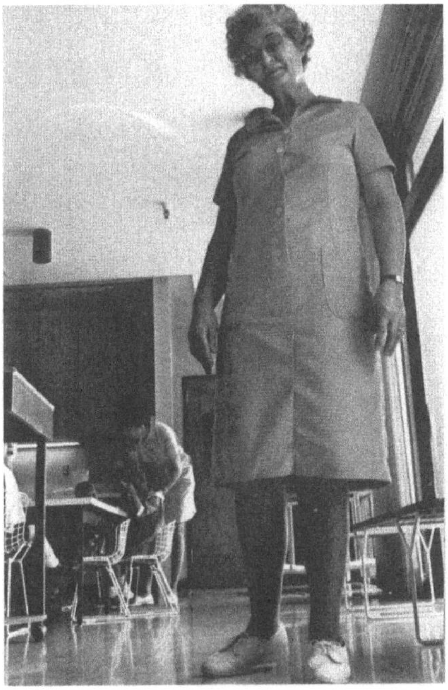

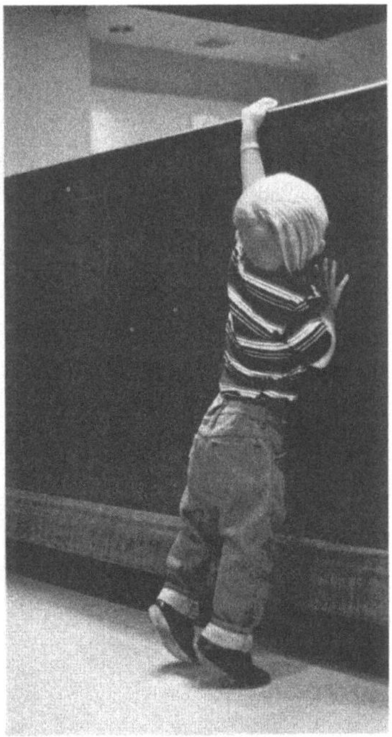

The size of a peer group will reflect the amount of emphasis placed on visual supervision, limited as it is by the distance one can see, as well as the importance given to maintaining a personal relation between the child and one or two adults. Both the size of the peer group and the number of different adults the child comes into contact with have particular importance for toddlers, as this is the time they learn to talk. Developmental psychologists have shown that exposure to too many persons, all with different ways of talking — often not the child's primary language — retards a young child's speech development.

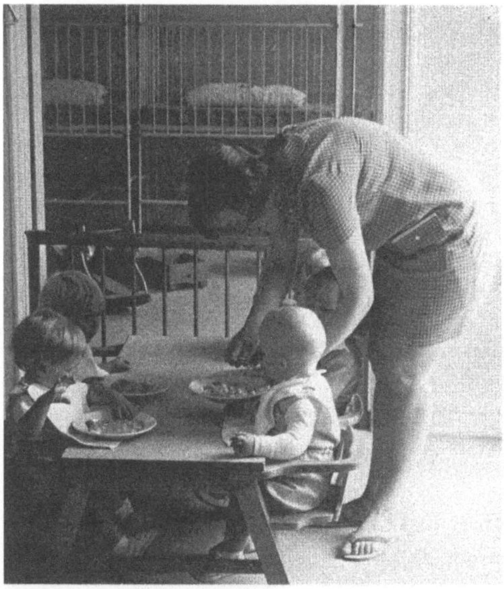

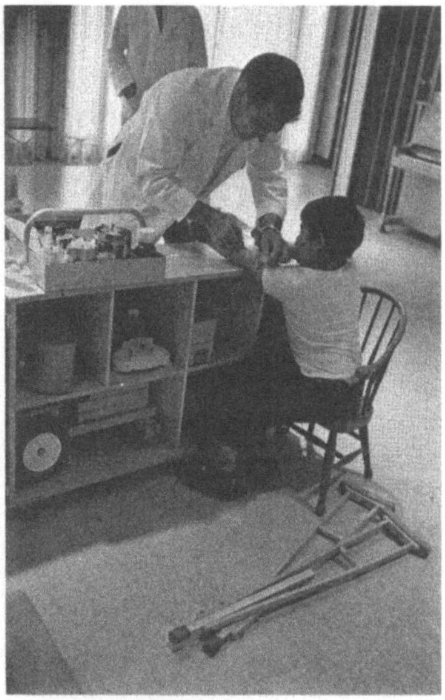

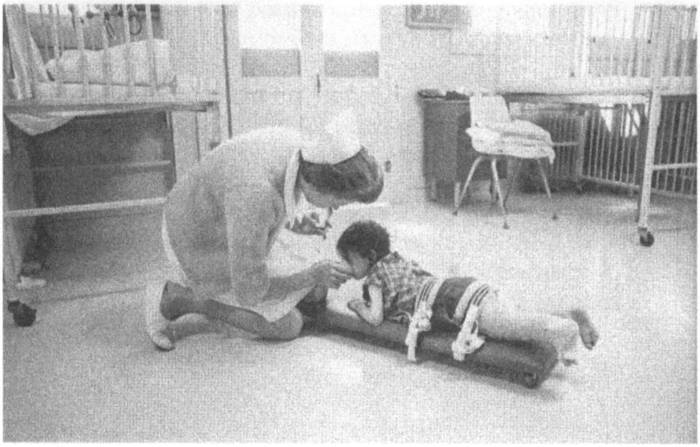

## *Design Guidelines*

Design raised platform areas for eating and playing so that children can be comfortably seated with their feet on the floor, while the nurse can still help them without straining her back by bending.

Provide raised tubs for bathing young children.

Use electric beds and cribs that can be easily raised and lowered, placing the mattress at an appropriate height for nurses' work.

Design the playroom or multipurpose room with a high ceiling over the central portion, and low ceiling heights in adjacent alcoves. Adults look smaller if the ceiling is higher, and lower ceiling alcoves provide cozy places for children to play.

Design balconies over the alcoves. Children can thus have another vantage point for viewing the world and can look down on the adults. If balconies are well screened, there is no danger of falling.

Lower window sills so that children can see out. Locate special windows at different heights for the specific use of children of different sizes.

Use child-size sinks and toilets.

Hang mirrors so that children can see themselves without climbing.

Provide hanging space within reach of children so they can learn to put away their own things.

Design the floor to serve as a play and work surface. The floor should be warm, easily cleaned, and covered with different textures to identify special areas, such as for play or work.

Provide lighting near the floor adequate for looking at pictures, drawing, and for other close activities, because children use the floor as a table.

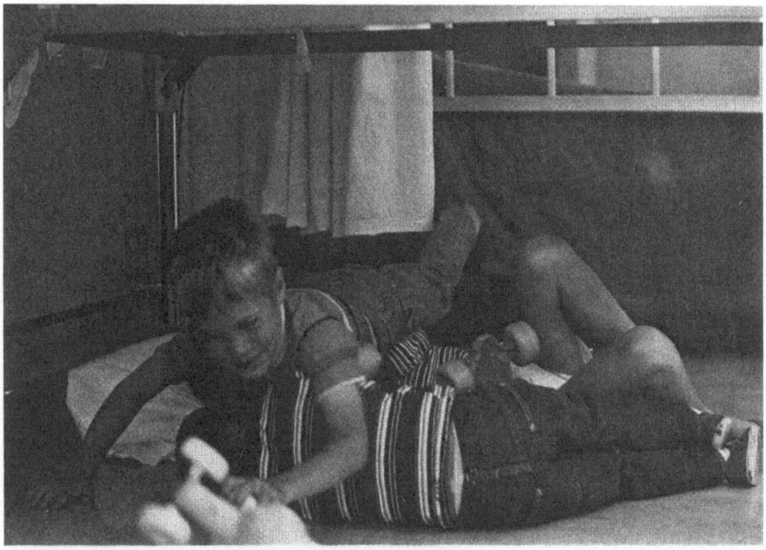

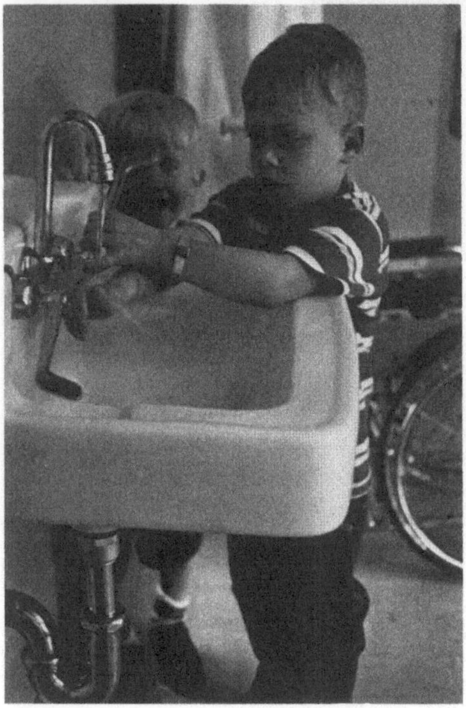

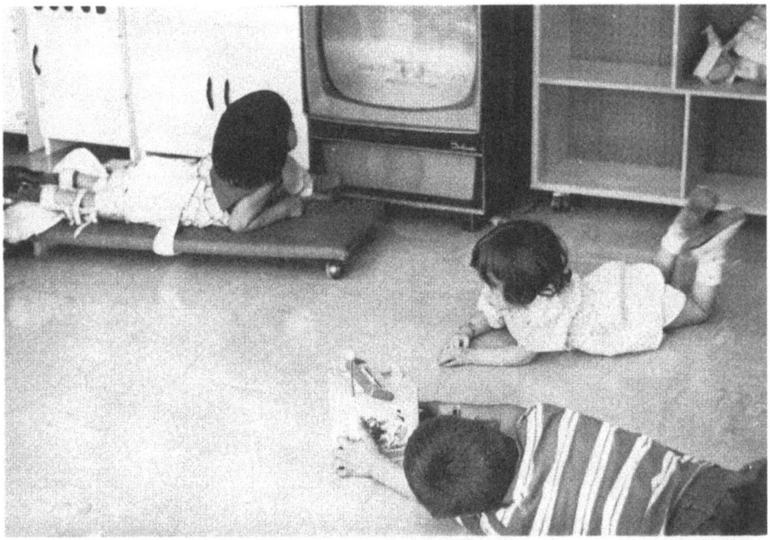

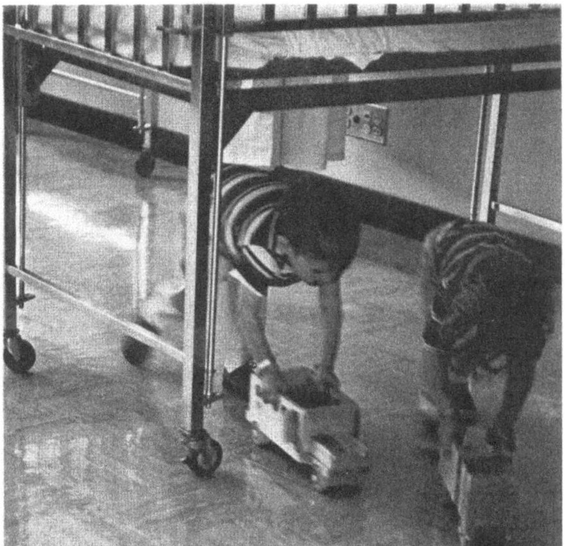

## Promote Autonomy and Independence



Between the ages of one and five the young child develops skills in eating, washing, dressing, and controlling bowel and bladder function. In the hospital setting it is far easier to be fed, washed, dressed, and toileted than to assume responsibility for one's own care. This is certainly true of adults. Much has been written about the so-called "stripping process," in which the adult patient is stripped both of his clothing and the ability to care for himself.[9] For a child to continue to care for himself is doubly difficult. The child's slowness and messiness as he helps himself upset tight hospital routines and often do not meet hospital hygiene standards for cleanliness.

A child often reacts to hospitalization with regressive behavior. To counter this, the staff must make great efforts to help him continue to develop his autonomy and independence. The physical setting must make it easy for a child to feed himself, wash, dress, and go to the toilet.

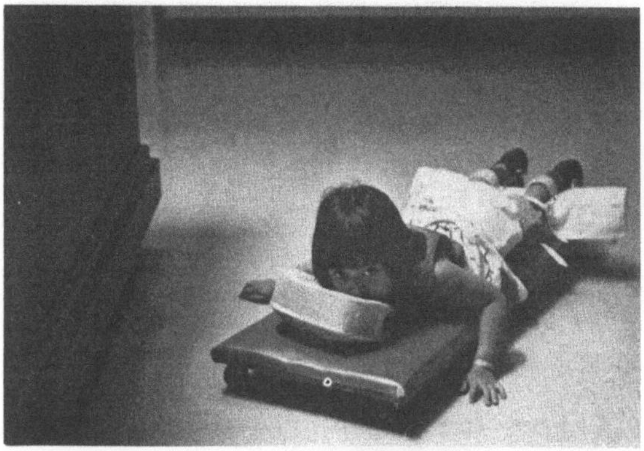

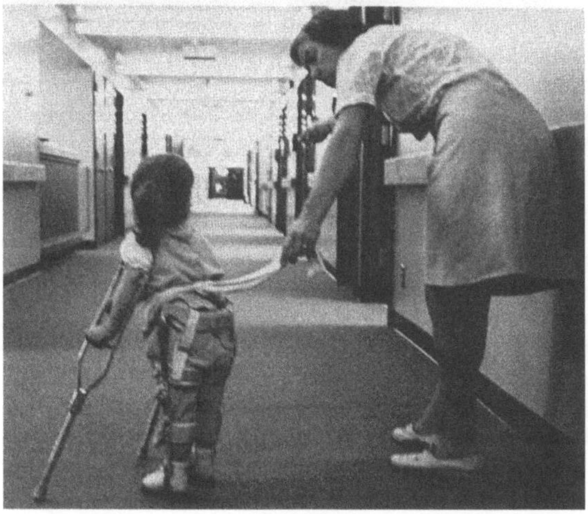

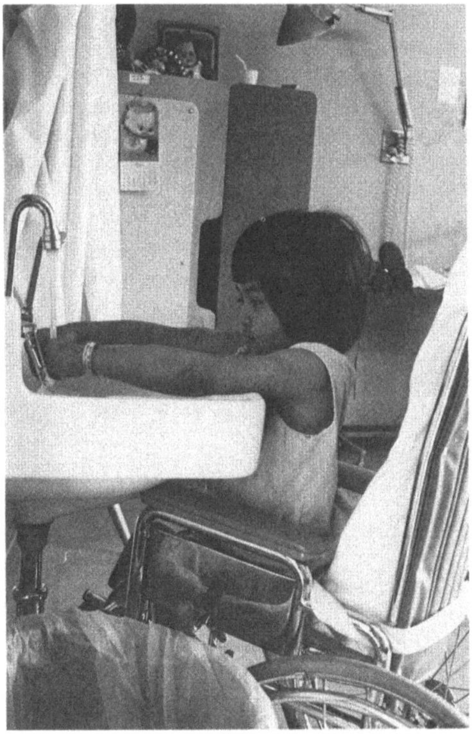

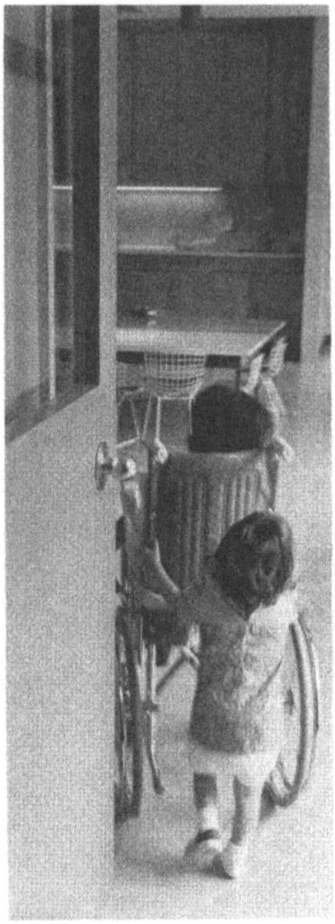

EATING

Children often eat poorly in the hospital. Learning to eat is a messy experience under the best possible conditions. Children do spill and throw food as they experiment with its tactile qualities.

Eating is a learning experience that requires staff patience. "Comfortable seating is also a part of the teaching situation. The child as well as the meal should be well balanced." [10] The hospital has special problems in providing appropriate environments for children in casts, on gurneys, and in bed.

*Design Guidelines*

Make eating a quiet social time. Place children together, whether they are in wheelchairs, gurneys, or can be up at their tables. Provide high chairs and feeding tables for toddlers.

Make the floor in the eating area easy to clean so that spilled food can be cleaned up with minimum fuss.

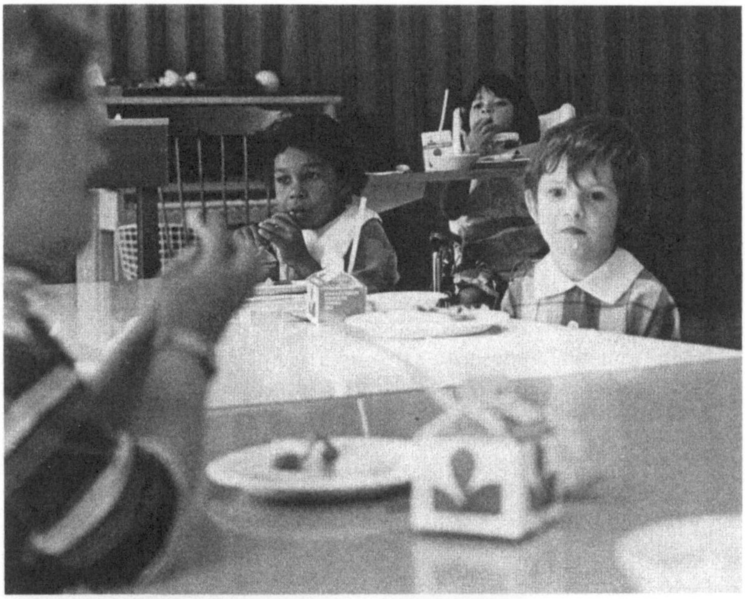

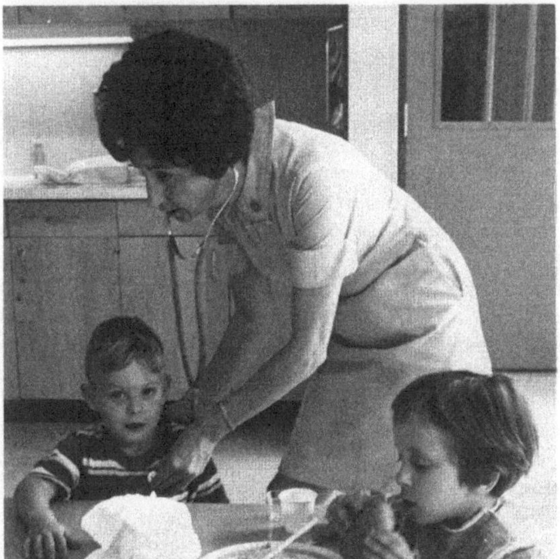

WASHING FACILITIES

Part of a child's devolpment is the gradual assumption of responsibility for his own body. Eventually children learn to wash their own faces and hands and to brush their own teeth.

*Design Guidelines* Provide low washbasins and adequate clearance underneath for juvenile wheelchairs.

CLOTHING STORAGE

Young children do not have large numbers of personal possessions, but it is important that they have their own identifiable places so as to safeguard their belongings.

*Design Guidelines* Design a small but private place for each child in which to store his clothing and belongings.

TOILETING

Gradually, but not without difficulty, the child masters his body and his bodily functions. By two years most children are physiologically capable of controlling their bowel and bladder sphincters, but how they use this new ability depends on whether they think of it in time, and if they feel like it.[11] Hospitalized children commonly regress in bowel and bladder control. This kind of regression takes place not only in the hospital but anywhere that emotional stress is high and the environment new.

A young child may need help in learning to use a strange bathroom. "It sometimes happens that a child around 2 has become so well trained to his own potty chair or toilet seat that he can't perform anywhere else. You can't urge or scold him into it. He will probably wet his pants eventually." [12]

Nursing personnel learn to handle this problem in a matter-of-fact, neutral sort of way, and to clean up the mess quietly and with no disapproval. Explaining the facilities to the child sometimes helps; so does learning his language for toileting.

Because of their lack of control, young children need easy and immediate access to the toilet. An observation about nursery schools is also true of the hospital: "Although architects and those responsible for planning the nursery school building should know that two-year-old children have to get to the toilet often, they seem to be oblivious . . . this

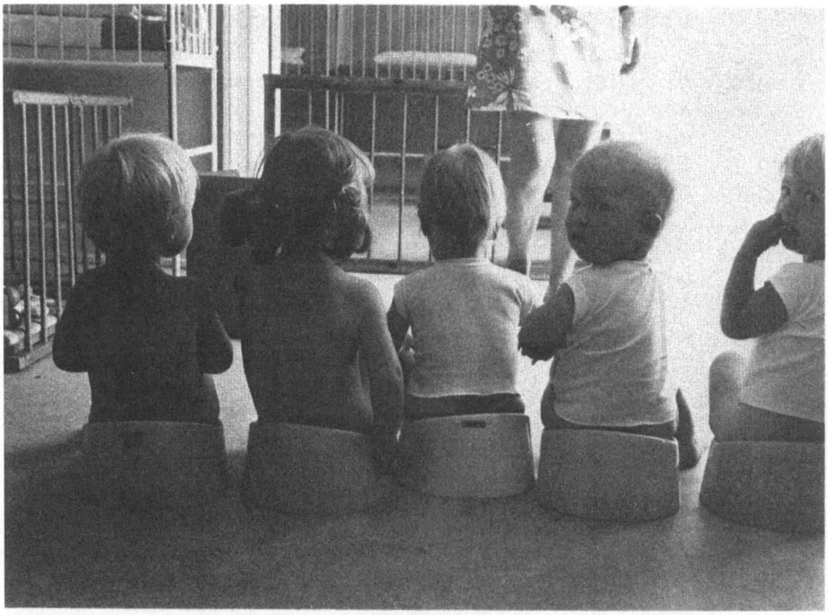

feature . . . more than any other architectural arrangement affects the pupil-teacher arrangement possible in a given set-up." [13]

The child's different perspective should also be taken into account: "Whatever *we* may think of the convenience and efficiency of indoor plumbing, the small child has his own ideas. This vitreous monster with its yawning jaws does not invite friendship or confidence at this age. The most superficial observation will reveal that it swallows up objects with a mighty roar, causes them to disappear in its secret depths, then rises again thirstily for its next victim which might be — just anyone." [14]

*Design Guidelines*

Make toilets visible, easily accessible, and adjacent to indoor and outdoor play areas, as young children need to use the toilet at a moment's notice.

Provide for potty chair (even a child's own) as well as water closets. The water closets should be both small scale and adult size, with silent plumbing.

Make the toilet area visible to the nurses. Privacy is generally not a problem for young children, and an easily visible toilet area reduces the need for supervisory personnel.

## Provide Challenges and Stimulation

A challenging, stimulating environment for toddlers and preschoolers is one that presents opportunities for him to explore the natural world and the human one, to develop and test skills, to develop physical coordination and strength, and to engage in dramatic, imaginative ideas. Children in this age group find their challenge and stimulation largely through play.

Play has been characterized as "the child's work." Through play, the child develops his skills, acts out his fears, and learns how to relate to other human beings. All children play as part of their normal activity. Moreover, the entire purpose of the hospital can also be conveyed to the child through play.[15]

A toddler's motor performance is polished by constant and enthusiastic practice. Observers of toddlers' behavior comment on their indomitable urge to exercise emerging skills. "The reason the 18-month-old is always on the go is that he just found he can go." [16]

The toddler plays largely by himself, with occasional glances at a playmate. At one, a child will play with others when they initiate simple games; if another rolls a ball at him, he will roll it back. By three, he plays both independently and with others. He is beginning to develop friendships with peers and to rely less on his primary relation with the family. He often attends kindergarten or nursery school, and begins to learn how to engage in dramatic play as he identifies with specific roles in playing house, fireman, astronaut, hospital, school, or store.

In addition, the content of the child's symbolic play derives from his experience, "which he shapes to suit his innermost needs. This is his way of understanding the things that happen to him — by reliving them in a simpler, safer, and more desirable form. Thus a child who has had an unpleasant encounter with the family doctor might play at being doctor, or both doctor and patient, in a situation somewhat removed from the pain of the actual experience and under his control . . . where an unpleasant reality is altered." [17] Many hospitals provide a limited repertoire of play opportunities, even though children and play are "infinitely varied and there is a need for an infinite variety of play opportunities." [18] Considerable imagination is necessary in the hospital, as the possibilities for play are constricted by a child's health and physical incapacity.

### INDOOR ACTIVITY SPACE

At the turn of the century, play space for hospitalized toddlers and preschoolers was thought of as a luxury; now it is known to be a necessity. Preschool children need special play areas adapted to their special needs. The American Academy of Pediatrics states that for children in hospitals: "a playroom with an adequate supply of toys, books, and games is not a luxury or a place where beds may be placed in an emergency. It is a therapeutic adjunct for convalescent and ambulatory patients. It is a necessary part of every pediatric unit." [19]

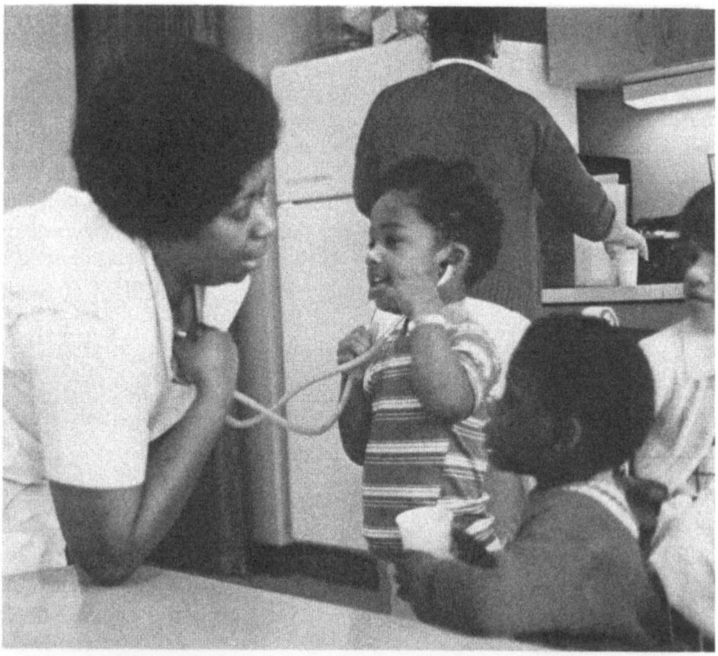

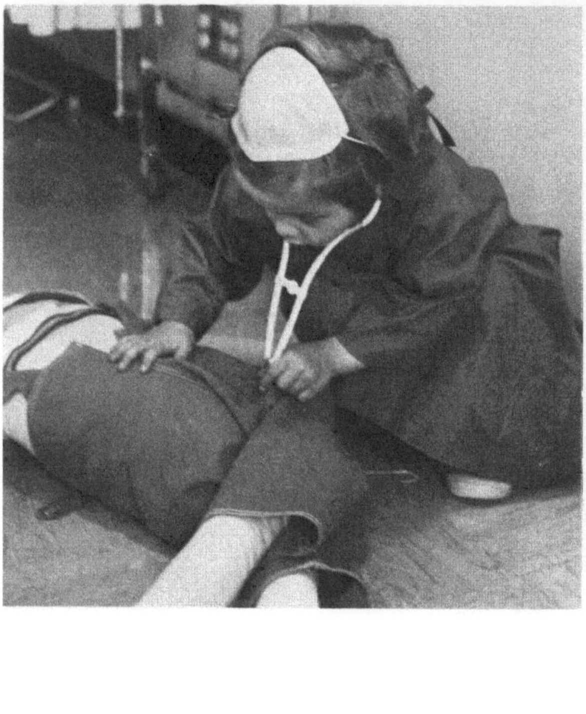

The indoor activities area must serve several purposes. It is at once the place for building with blocks, painting, acting out roles, and music. Often it also serves as an eating place or a place for visiting parents. Much work has been done on the design of nursery school areas that have similar activities. The problem that makes hospital design difficult is the need to accommodate patients in beds, on gurneys, in cribs, in wheelchairs, or on flex boards.

One can approach the development of play areas in the hospital in several ways. One approach is to make the sleeping areas large enough for play to take place in these areas and to include children confined to bed.[20] Another approach is to promote separate play areas and design

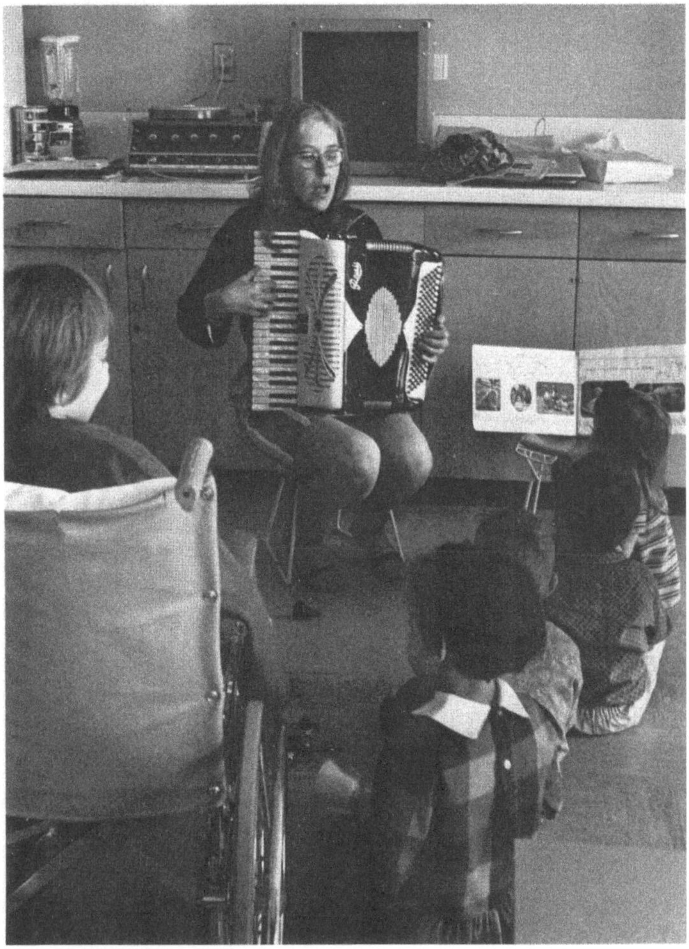

them so as to accommodate children in cribs, gurneys, and wheelchairs. "The space should not be too big, as it is in a school gymnasium or auditorium. No homelike or practical placing of equipment can be made in such a vast place, which only suggests running and vigorous noisy play to the children." [21]

## *Design Guidelines*

Connect the play area with an outdoor area at the same level. Adults should be able to supervise visually both indoor and outdoor areas from either indoors or outdoors.

Adjoin the play area to a toilet that is accessible without opening doors.

Provide a kitchenette for snacks, juice, and other food.

Make the floor warm and soft. The part of the floor area used for eating should be easily cleaned.

Design alcoves for different activities going on at the same time, including parent observation.

Build adequate storage facilities for supplies that a child can reach.

Provide a sink for messy play, low enough for children to use, plus another one high enough for adults.

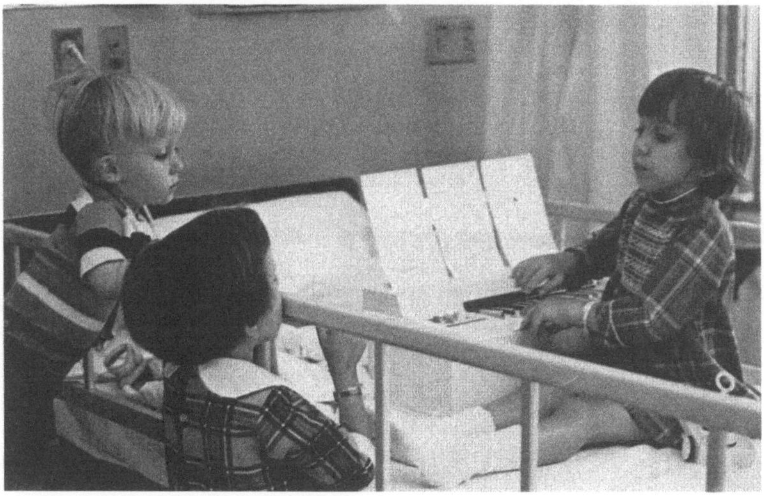

OUTDOOR ACTIVITY SPACE

The playground must offer "some challenge to the most skillful child . . . and some opportunity for successful achievement to the least skillful." [22] Outdoor facilities for children in hospitals are relatively new. Older hospitals in urban areas rarely have even a play roof for the pediatric unit. Even in less dense situations the use of the outside has been neglected. With earlier ambulation, and with the change in disease patterns from fever and contagion to metabolic, respiratory, and congenital problems, the need for outdoor play areas for pediatric units has become accepted. The Platt Report states: "Children who are in bed need a view and facilities for outside play whether on a balcony or a playground." [23] The Nuffield Foundation studies on planning facilities for children in hospitals state, "Whatever the shape of the building, it ought to open onto a garden or courtyard for the children's use." [24]

The design of a play area for hospitalized young children need not differ basically from play areas for healthy prekindergarten children, with the obvious exception that it must also provide specialized opportunities for play by children on gurneys, in wheelchairs, and in casts. In either case, "planning a playground for children aged two to six calls for more than an equipment catalogue." [25] It should provide for different kinds and levels of skills. Opportunities must be provided for the hospitalized child who may be restricted in any of numerous ways in the kind of activity he can perform. Emphasis should be placed on providing space and equipment conducive to quiet creative and make-believe play.

## *Design Guidelines*

Locate the outdoor play area directly adjacent to the indoor play area. An easily accessible and supervisable outdoor area will be used more frequently than one in a remote location, requiring specially planned and supervised excursions.

Design indoor and outdoor play areas on the same level, because children in wheelchairs or on gurneys and crutches cannot easily manage changes in level.

Combine ground surfaces so that children can wheel toys, dig, play with water, and ride bikes. The ground surfaces should be nonabrasive, such as indoor-outdoor carpet or grass.

Allow for sun or shade, depending on what is most desirable for the particular climate or the region.

Make it possible for staff to supervise all parts of the outdoor play area from inside the playroom.

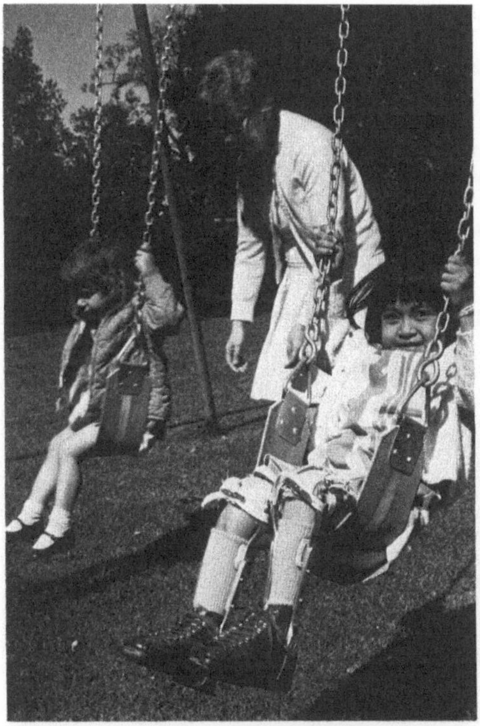

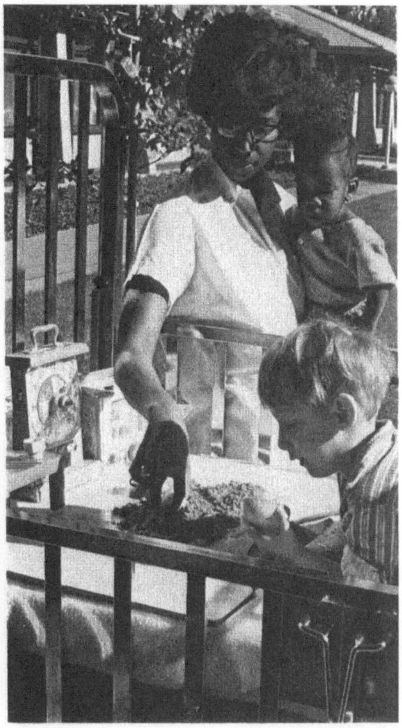

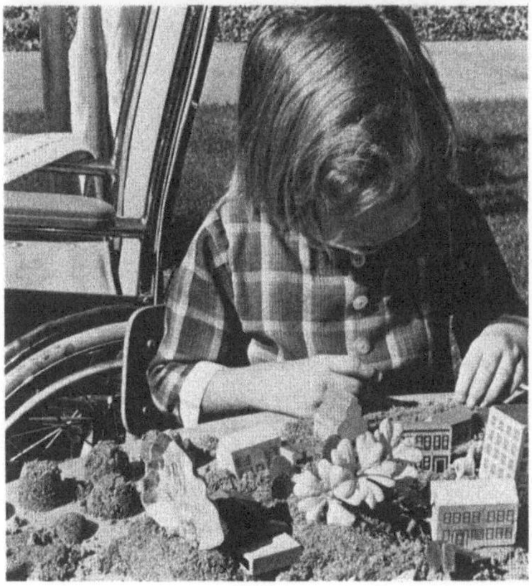

Supply soft surfaces under all climbing equipment.

Supply a hose, wading pool, and opportunity for water play.

Grade with gentle inclines for running and peddling. Add grass mounds and humps and bridges that can be used from above and below.

Plant trees and shrubs around the edges to avoid obstructing the visibility necessary for supervision.

Provide opportunities to garden.

Build storage shelter for toys and yard equipment.

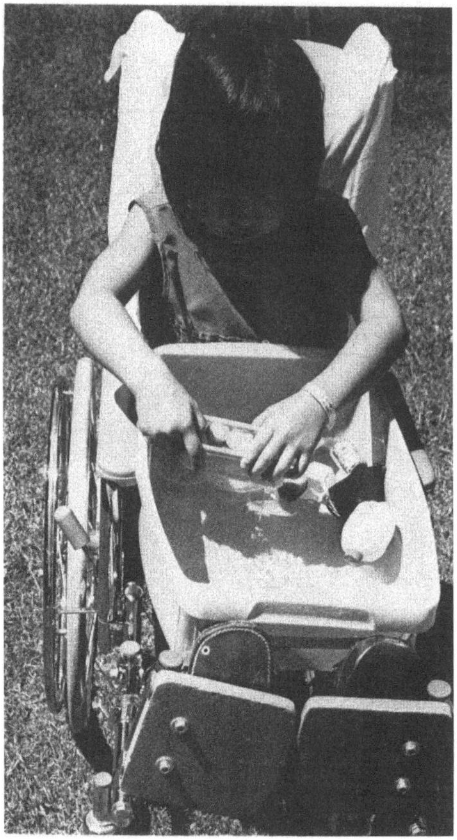

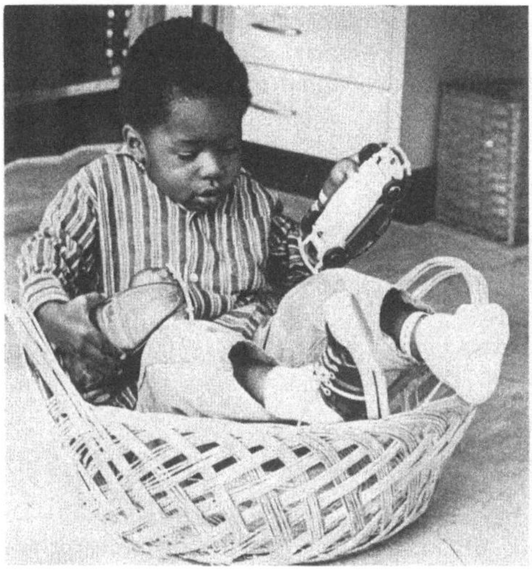

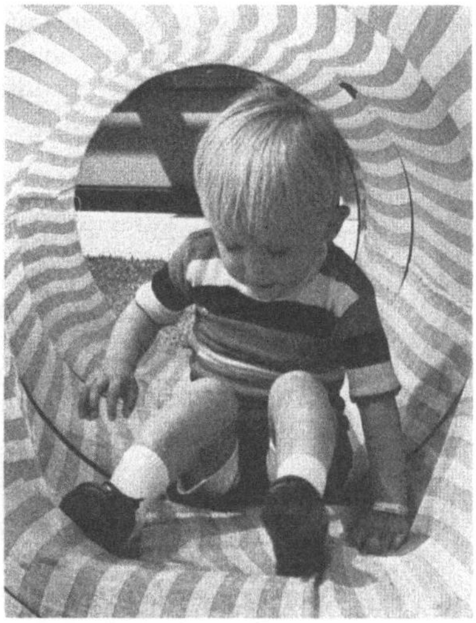

MATERIALS AND EQUIPMENT

A distinguishing characteristic of young children's spontaneous activities is that they involve materials briefly used, for a variety of purposes. A study of the use of play materials by nursery school children showed that the children spent 98 percent of their time in play with materials.[26]

The materials children seek out vary at different age levels. "Once the child becomes capable of appreciating the effects of his own actions on different materials, trying these out seems to follow 'automatically,' limited only by his skill and the nature of the material." [27] There must be a variety of materials, including those that can be manipulated, like mud, water, sand, and starch; those that can be built with, like blocks, boards, and boxes; those that are props for dramatic play, like stethoscopes and syringes. "Fingerpaints, soft clay, and wet sand have the natural advantage of bringing the child in direct contact with his medium with no intervening tool." [28]

Children prefer to play in environments that they can manipulate and change. They prefer malleable materials that they themselves can organize.[29] Among the most versatile play materials, along with blocks, are crates and empty cartons. Children love to climb into crates and cartons, and if these are not available, they will sometimes use empty shelves for the purpose. "Cosy places seem to offer an area of safety from a threatening world." [30] Emma Plank has observed that battered children gravitate toward the security of a small place when they first come to the hospital.

Some hospitals use plants and animals in their playrooms. Great care must be exercised in their choice, as both plants and animals can cause allergic reactions and carry disease. It is possible to develop a nonallergenic zoo of fish, snakes, lizards, iguanas, and salamanders, but many children are not used to these animals and even find them fearful.

*Design Guidelines*

Provide opportunities to use a variety of manipulable materials.

Provide clothing and props allowing children to imitate doctors, nurses, firemen, pilots, and other adult roles.

Provide blocks and boxes for children to develop their own hideaways.

BATHING AND WATER PLAY

"To an adult, water may mean only washing and drinking. To a child, it means at least washing, drinking, and play. Where no provision is made for water play, children are likely to make shift with the washing and drinking arrangements, flooding the bathroom and stopping up the drinking fountain." [31]

In the hospital setting, water offers play opportunities, even for especially weak or physically handicapped children. Some hospitals provide water play for children in wheelchairs and in bed. Under these circumstances the extent of water play is both limited and hard on nurses. Beds and children have to be changed, floors mopped, and equipment dried.

The logical setting for water play in the hospital environment is the bath. For small children, bathing is an enjoyable social function. It should be possible to provide for both bathing and water play in a specially designed room equipped for this purpose, even though exceptional antiseptic standards are necessary.

*Design Guidelines*

Put bathtubs for young children in specially designed rooms associated with play areas rather than with toilet facilities.

Place several tubs adjacent to one another for parallel bathing.

Develop an image of the hospital bath as a spa, a Roman bath, rather than as an aseptic tub.

Provide additional raised water areas where children in gurneys and wheelchairs can sail boats and take care of indoor gardens. Sinks should be easily available. Wading pool, hose, and sprinklers should be outside.

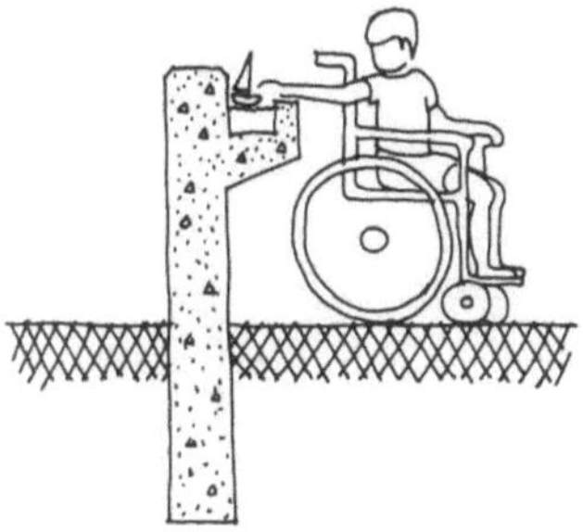

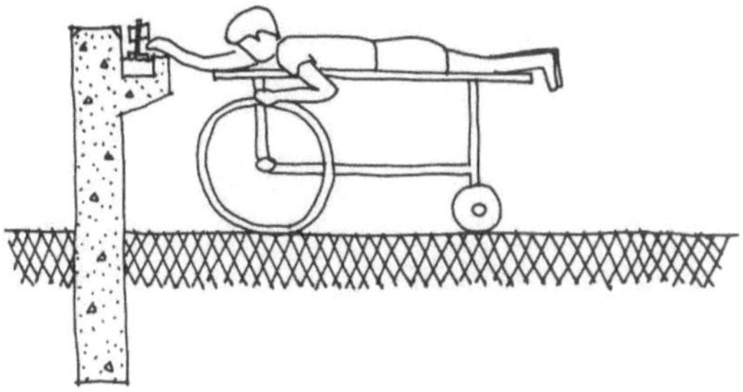

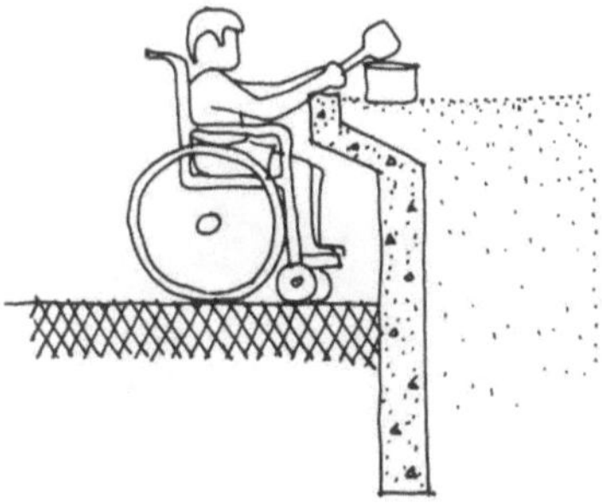

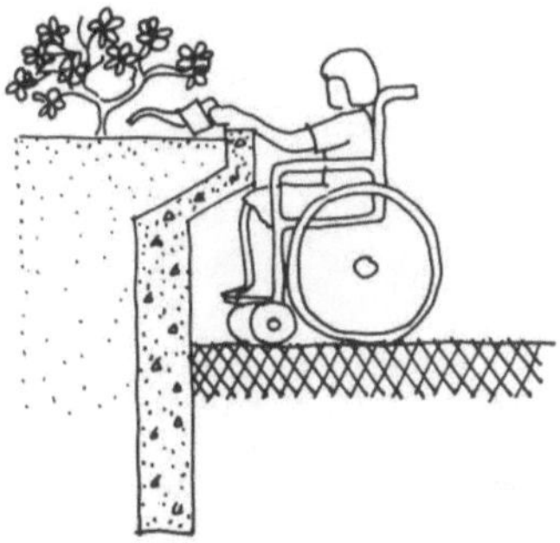

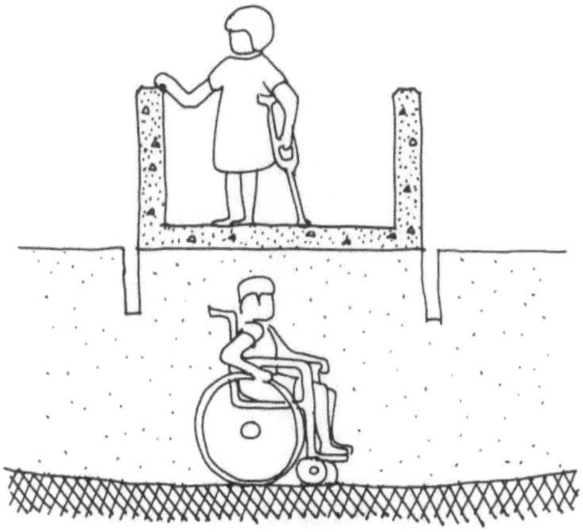

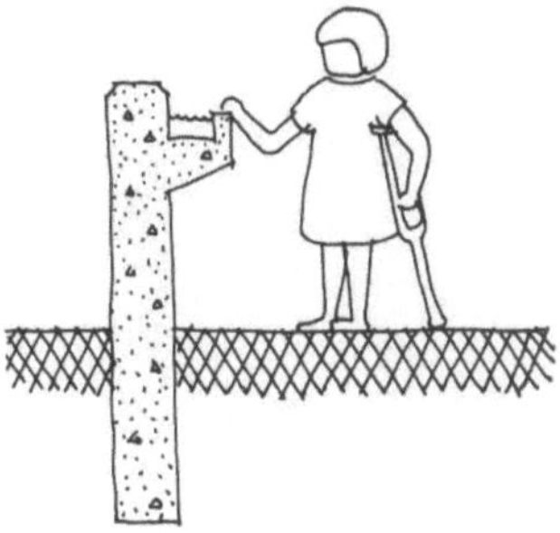

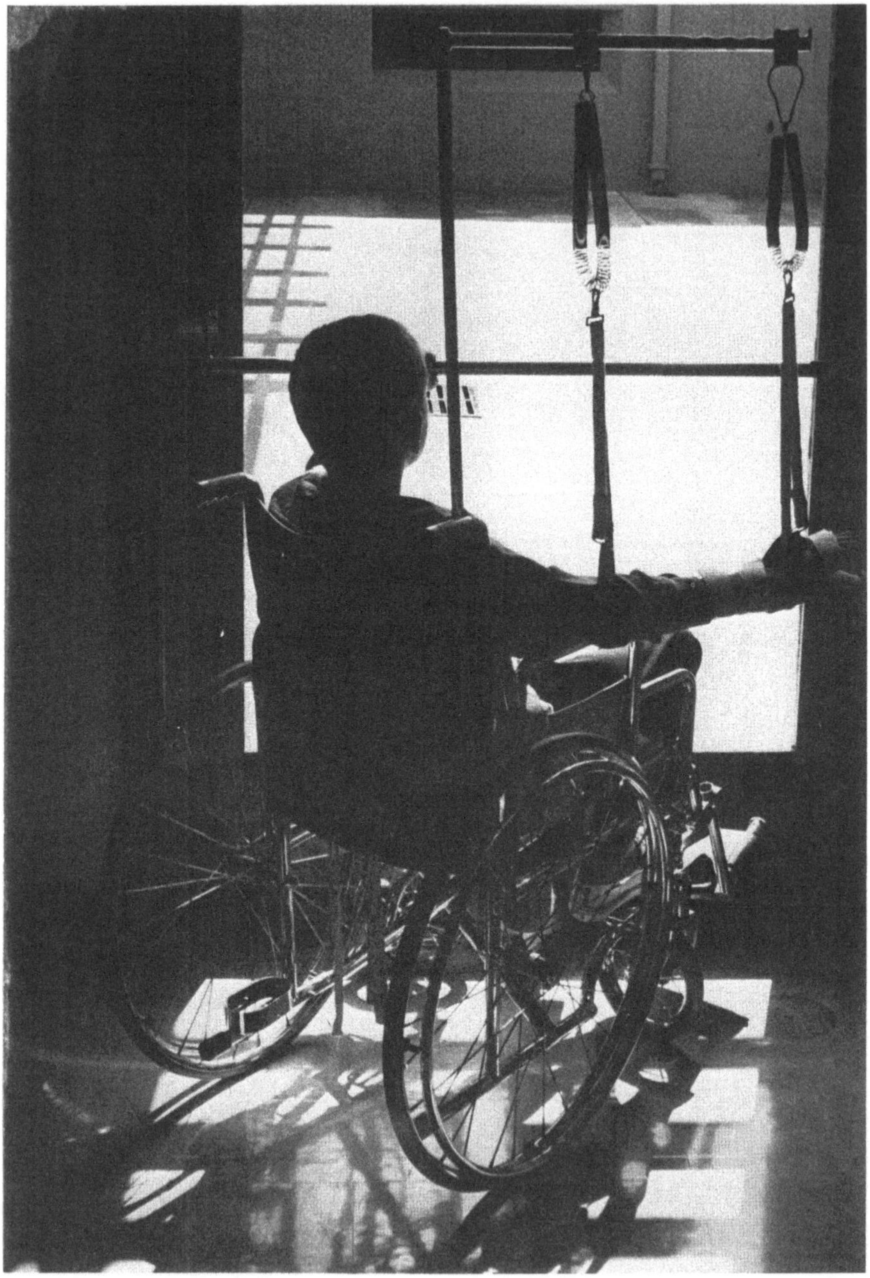

# Grade School Children 5

The growth of the grade school child (6–12 years) is slow and even, up to the preadolescent growth spurt. During these middle years the child is sick less often than as a younger child. He is less susceptible to accidents and requires much less careful supervision than do toddlers and preschool children. He has not yet developed the adolescent's persistent questioning of authority and open rebelliousness. Psychologists call this stage the latency period, a time during which the child shows little overt interest in sexual concerns and works to develop a variety of skills necessary for eventual independence from the family. However, "because of his desire for independence he may be irritating to his parents and present a problem in discipline." [1]

Jean Piaget has termed this period of mastering important skills the stage of concrete operations of thought and interpersonal relations.[2] Mollie and Russell Smart have described this age as one in which the child begins to relate things and ideas: "he operates on (does something to) objects, ideas and symbols. He adds and subtracts. He classifies and orders. He applies rules to social situations. Each operation fits into a system, and the systems fit together." [3]

The grade school child develops from the awkward preschool child to a person capable of considerable motor coordination, practicing this skill in athletic games and a variety of crafts. He forms his first close mutual friendships and learns to work in teams. Often he prefers friends of his own sex, with the influence of his peers rivaling the influence of his parents and other adults. In developing social relations, he learns to accept and modify social and moral rule systems. He enjoys dramatizing his concept of social rules and roles through dressing and play-acting. Finally, the grade school child learns to express himself verbally, to write, and to read. He acquires the basic concepts of number, weight, space, time, and speed.

The characteristics of the child during preadolescent years, although often ignored by psychologists in favor of the more dramatic and enigmatic characteristics of other age groups, more accurately predict his adult psychological health than do those during either the upheavals of adolescence or his earlier years.[4] One task of the hospital, therefore, must be to provide an environment that will allow the child to develop and practice the wide range of physical, social, and cognitive skills that he needs eventually to achieve independence from adults. For the grade school child, hospitalization poses a threat of continued and regressive dependency and of falling behind in the development of basic skills, especially as measured in the grade school. Coupled with this threat is a continuing fear of mutilation and anxiety produced by the unknown and frightening aspects of the hospital environment.

The ways in which illness and hospitalization affect latency-age children relate directly to the developmental tasks specific to this period of life. Lucie Jessner, observing the reactions of sick children in latency, has described the effects of illness at this age on ego functions, body image, and family relations.[5] She points out that, whereas the healthy school-age child takes his body for granted, illness produces a heightened and uncomfortable concern about physiological functions and forces the child to cope prematurely with concepts of illness and death. Motor restriction limits his ability to maintain his newly developed sense of mastery through physical activity. Threats to body intactness especially affect boys, involving their concern about masculinity. The image of parents as benevolent guardians is challenged by reality when the sick child sees his parents helpless to protect him from suffering. He may even imgaine that he is being punished for misdeeds, by being hospitalized and separated from the warmth and support of his family. The sick child reacts to these real and imagined situations with increased dependency, regression, and anxiety.

Nonetheless, children in this age group probably cope more ably with hospitalization than do either younger or older children. They can usually understand and accept the necessity of their hospitalization. In a study of two hundred hospitalized children between two and twelve years of age, Dane Prugh and his coauthors found the lowest incidence of immediate, severe reactions in the six-to-twelve-year-old group. Although the early latency-age child still commonly manifested anxiety, fewer children showed panic reactions or reactions to parental separation. The children of this age group characteristically attached their feelings of anxiety to potentially painful or frightening experiences, and they demonstrated more restless and compulsive behavior than did younger children.[6] In another study in which six-to-nine-year-old children were interviewed in the hospital, they expressed attitudes of passive conformity and the need to win recognition by being productive.[7]

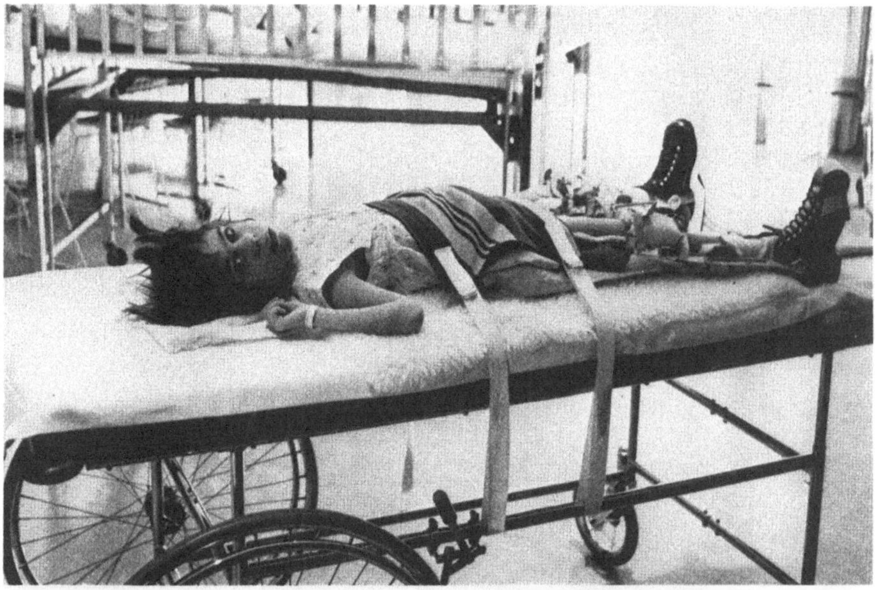

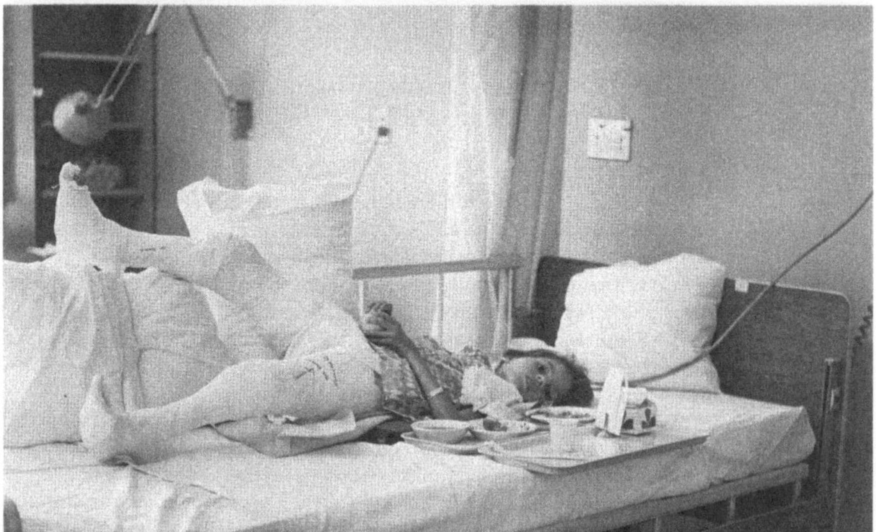

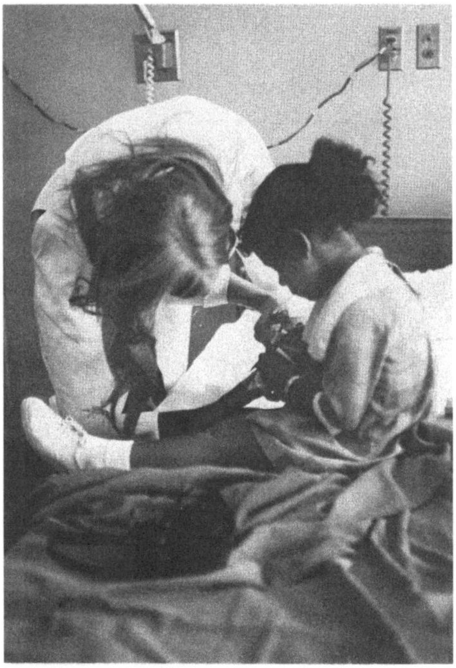

## Provide Continuity in Acquiring and Exercising Cognitive and Motor Skills

### SCHOOLROOM

The grade school child's acquisition of skills as measured by schoolwork is very important to him. Moreover, when such children are hospitalized, they are concerned about all the extra work they must face after returning to their regular school. Falling behind is discouraging and can precipitate serious learning problems. A suitably equipped hospital school setting will therefore assist children in keeping up with schoolwork even if they are confined to bed or a wheelchair and even if they are some distance from their home school.

Yet children often find the lessons offered in the hospital to be irrelevant, earning no credit in their real school or social setting. One boy of ten years old, for example, who was in the hospital for the repair of a hernia, resisted schooling for a week, informing the hospital teacher that he would do real schoolwork at school but that he certainly would not do the hospital's work which was not going to count at the real school. In contrast, in the Hospital School at Canton, Massachusetts, the children who could not be moved into the classroom, even on gurneys, were able to participate in class discussions via closed-circuit TV, and they found this a much more involving educational experience than the short period of private tutoring possible each day at a similar cost.[8]

Eight to twelve students represent the greatest number of students that can be handled by one teacher if they require special personal attention. A survey of special classroom sizes in thirty-four large cities indicated a classroom size of about twelve students.[9] In a program where the child may spend only a few days or weeks, the classes should be smaller.

The hospital schoolroom can be a refuge from the medical environment and all it means in terms of treatments and pain.[10] At Children's Hospital at Stanford, the schoolrooms are located in a separate school building on the hospital grounds. They were designed by a specialist in school architecture, with aid from hospital specialists only to ensure correct placement of grab bars near blackboards and other details of design required for weakened or handicapped children. For the children, school is a different place from the hospital, and the day has more variety. One hospital teacher at Stanford University Medical Center stated that she finds it essential to maintain the classroom as a sanctuary from medical treatment. During the hours that children spend with her, they can relax. Each child's hours are scheduled so that treatments do not intrude on schooling.

Hospital rooms can be dreary and impersonal. It is thus easy for the child to avoid taking school seriously. At the same time, the child needs to be recognized for his successes and encouraged to continue his schoolwork.

## *Design Guidelines*

Provide electronic aides for keeping the child in touch with his home school and for keeping bed-bound or isolated children in touch with either hospital or home school. Telephones, closed-circuit TV, video tapes, and acoustic tapes all have their uses.

Provide enough space (600–1000 sq. ft.) in the hospital schoolroom to accommodate eight to twelve patients, some of whom will arrive on gurneys or in wheelchairs. Recommendations for classroom size vary widely, with larger dimensions being essential where patients are principally admitted for orthopedic treatment. For example, the California State School for cerebral palsied children uses 30′x40′ classrooms for grade school children. W. B. Schoenbohm suggests 24′x24′ as adequate for a hospital serving a wide variety of cases.[11]

Provide special aids so that weakened or handicapped children can participate more fully in the hospital schoolroom.

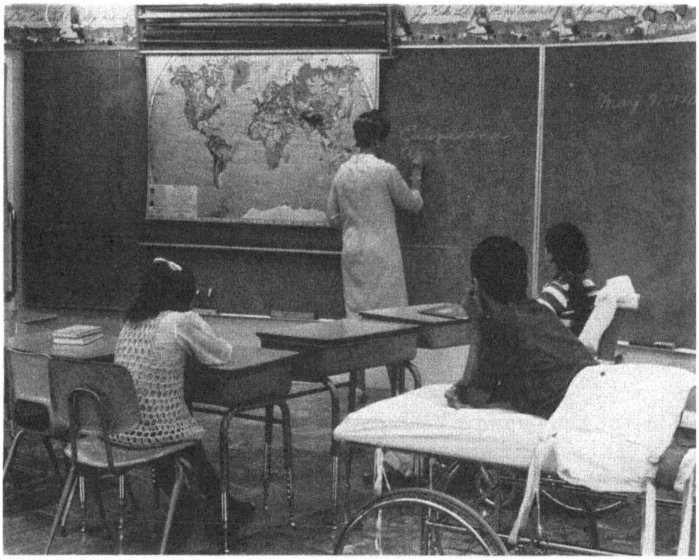

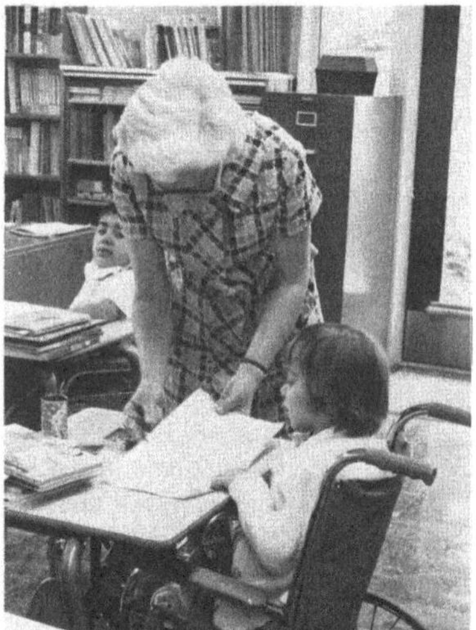

*Grade School Children*

These aids include grab bars near blackboards and painting easels, projecting blackboards for wheelchair use, and cantilevered low sinks for use with juvenile wheelchairs.

Provide generous amounts of display space for tacking up schoolwork and educational materials. One-third to one-half of the wall space should be tackable.

Locate the schoolroom in an area separate from the pediatric unit, not as a part of the medical environment.

### MUSIC PRACTICE ROOM

Grade school children first begin to explore music in a disciplined way through learning to play musical instruments. Playing these instruments would be an excellent way to fill the many hours in the hospital, as well as a therapeutic way to relax. Disabled or seriously ill children often find music to be one activity they can continue normally. Unfortunately, in many hospitals there is little possibility of finding a place where their music will not disturb others who are feeling ill.

*Design Guidelines*

Provide a soundproofed room suitable for music in grade school and adolescent units.

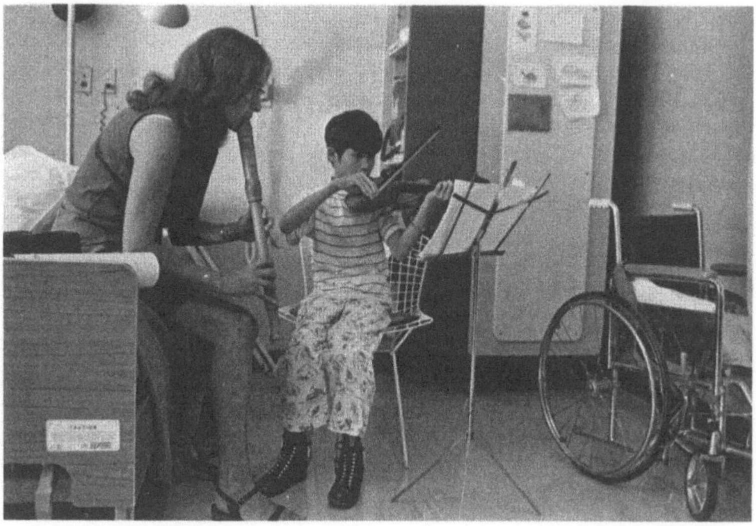

PLAY AND ATHLETICS AREA

Grade school children show an astonishing amount of energy. When healthy they bound from one activity to the next and sleep soundly at night. In the hospital, activity is restricted, and children do not always find it possible to get really tired — tired enough to sleep well. Yet many hospitalized children could engage in a variety of vigorous activities without danger, although these activities may not always be identical to those found on the grade school playground.[12]

Many of the suggestions for the preschool children's outdoor play area are directly relevant to hospitalized grade school children. The major difference is that grade school children have usually exhausted the possibilities of standard play equipment and enjoy group athletic and imaginative play more than do younger children. Adventure playgrounds, vacant lots, and other areas allowing creative participation and providing settings for a wide variety of imaginative play are popular with grade school children.

In the hospital, where many of these children have limitations on their mobility, emphasizing a variety of settings for creative and imaginative play is essential. Since much of the grade school child's outdoor play is highly imaginative, it depends on the use of a variety of settings.[13] It therefore demands more space than a tiny courtyard or balcony. A small space should not be tolerated if any alternative exists. In densely-built urban areas, even roof decks can be made acceptable through the use of outdoor carpeting, potted trees and plants, and other softening and space-dividing devices that enrich play opportunities.

Any playground should provide successes for all the children who play. Nothing discourages a child from needed physical activity so much as frequent and unrelieved failure.[14]

For activity in small groups, grade school children seek out places where a group can be together. This may be defined as a clubhouse, a fort, a ship, or any number of places. Children particularly value such places if they have participated to some degree in their construction. As R. D. Laing observed, "The two most important human needs are experience and control over one's own experience." [15]

## *Design Guidelines*

Provide a grade school outdoor play area with space for children who are moving on crutches, on gurneys, or in wheelchairs. In congested locations roofdecks might be acceptable for this purpose.

Provide activities that are possible for patients who are only partially mobile, such as basketball, tetherball, shuffleboard, horseshoe, or ring toss. Swimming, for many physically handicapped persons, provides a unique opportunity for physical freedom and exercise.

Provide materials for building clubhouses and other enclosed places. In the simplest case, this need be only huge cardboard cartons.

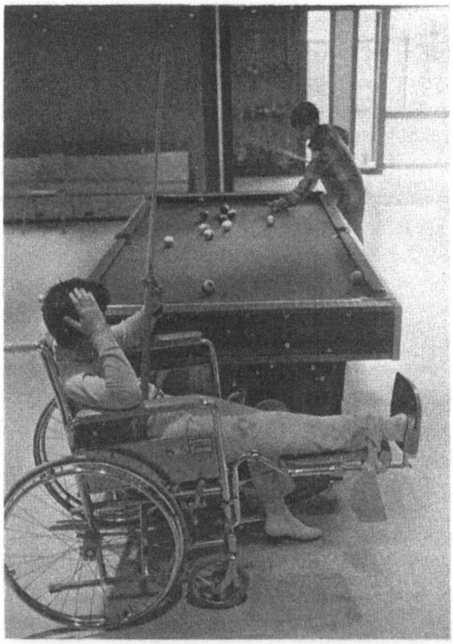

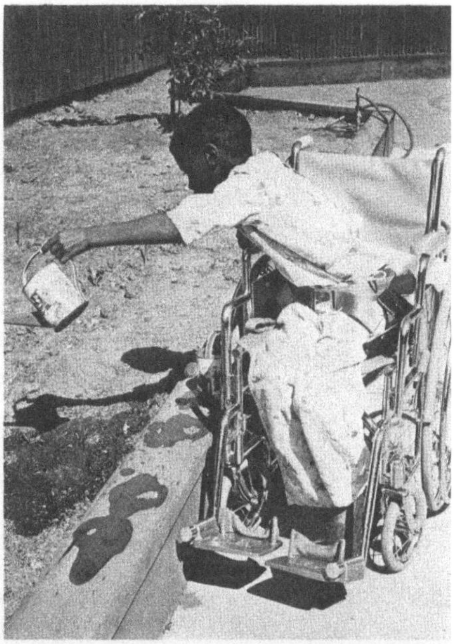

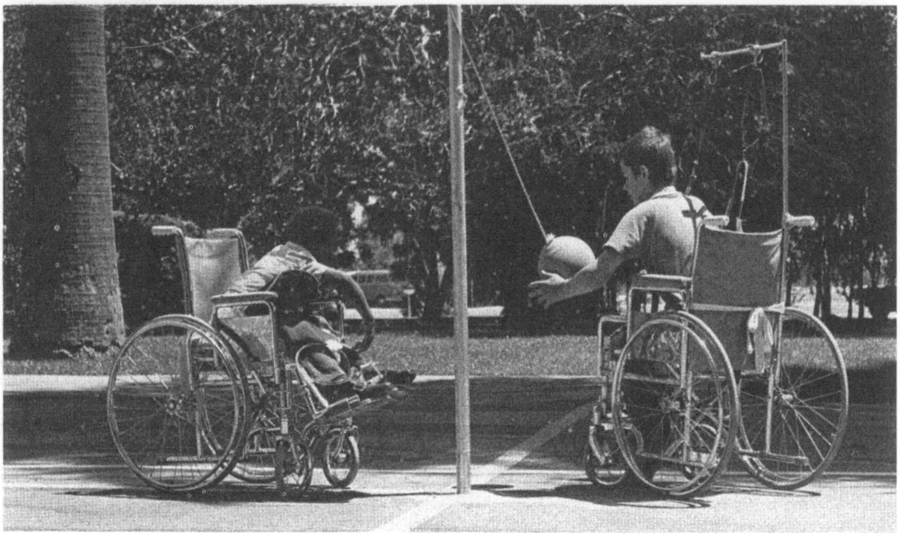

## Encourage Ability To Live and Work with Others

BEDROOM

During grade school years, children develop close, supportive friendships with children of the same sex. The sleeping environment can often reinforce these needed friendships in the hospital.

Although children do not always need to be sex-segregated, in Western culture they are more at home when sharing rooms with like-sexed siblings or friends. Nevertheless, during World War II, English children evacuated from London shared rooms with many other children, often in mixed-sex groups, without problems. In many other parts of the world siblings of mixed sexes share sleeping areas. In these instances, cultural patterns have been developed to handle the lack of physical privacy. For example, while living with migrant farm workers of Mexican descent, we observed that whole families who were forced to live in single rooms had developed nonspacial means of achieving modesty and privacy. Clothing was important for the former, quietness and politeness for the latter.[16] But the fact remains that in most parts of the United States mixed-sex groups of children older than seven or eight do not share the same sleeping area if it is avoidable. It is during this period that children develop body modesty.

Grade school children enjoy the company of several peers in small groups. Where four-bed rooms have been used, as at Children's Hospital at Stanford, they have been found to provide the children with companionship without being so large as to become boisterously uncontrollable.

The single over-the-bed table provided in a typical hospital room for eating, studying, and projects is insufficient for the bed-bound grade school child, whose projects may take days to complete and require many parts that are best stored on the work surface. It is annoying to have to clear away a complicated project every few hours for meal service. Children also display pictures of favorite athletes or movie stars, buttons, insects, models, and get-well cards from friends. One patient at a university medical center, a twelve-year-old boy with a severely fractured elbow, pointed with pride to the large number of letters received from his sixth-grade class. They were taped in rows on the wall in the only direction his traction would allow him to look comfortably. Although the tape was harmful to the wall enamel and was prohibited, the nursing staff gave priority to the boy's need to display his collection of letters.

### *Design Guidelines*

Provide separate bedrooms for boys and girls.

Provide multibed rooms accommodating about four children.

Provide a project space near each bed. Include in it a surface for studying and making things and a place to store project materials. The project space for each bed will vary with the mobility of the patient. An ambulant patient may use the multipurpose space. Bed-bound patients will obviously need more space for projects near their beds.

Provide space for displaying collections, get-well cards, and art work. A steel wall surface with magnetic tacks is one hygienic solution.

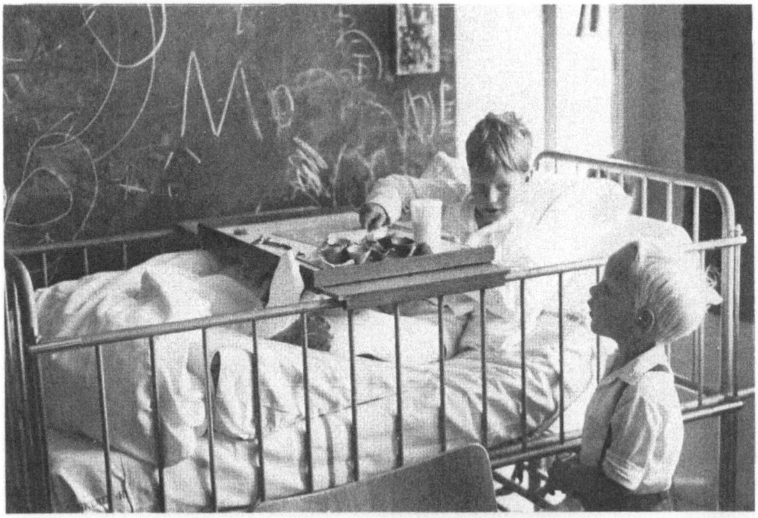

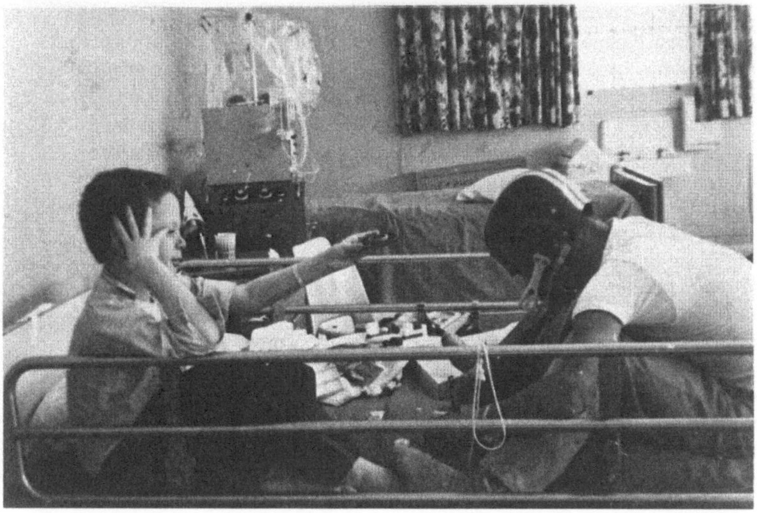

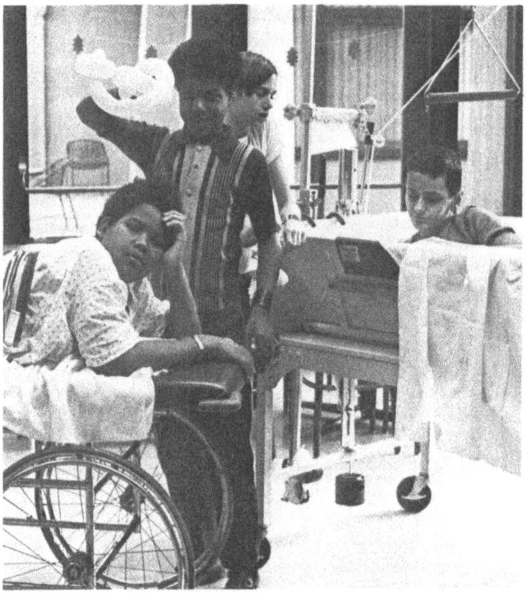

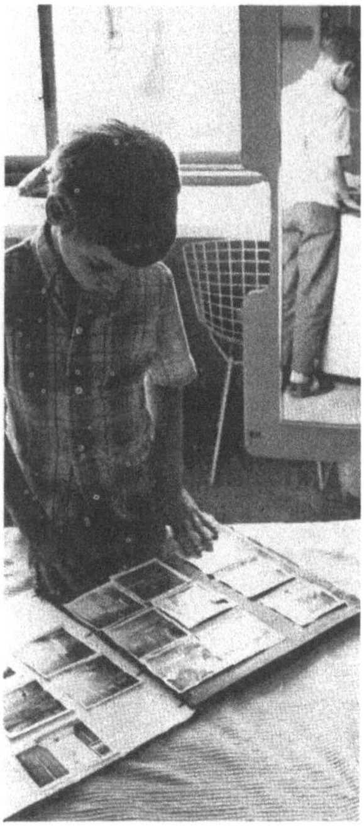

MULTIPURPOSE SPACE

Healthy grade schoolers are constantly busy, actively exploring their physical environment and pursuing a variety of projects and games. They collect and make a wide array of objects. They engage in sports, table games, and card games, often delighting in measuring their performance against that of a parent or other adult. They dress up and perform impromptu dramatic events as well as practiced plays. The multiplicity of activities suggests the need for an adaptable space within which small groups of grade school girls or boys can pursue their chosen activities freely.

In Children's Hospital at Stanford, sixteen grade school patients use about 400 square feet of multipurpose space, which is also used as a dining area. This provision seems adequate, since separate school rooms and occupational therapy rooms are available. Sixteen children seems a manageable number. It has also been suggested that family living and dining areas should be enlarged by encircling them with project alcoves. These alcoves would be undisturbed by meals and visiting and could even be screened off if the project was messy and not up to housekeeping standards for a formal living area.[17]

Boys and girls often want to put up a wall between their activities. A room may be claimed exclusively by one sex group or the other unless

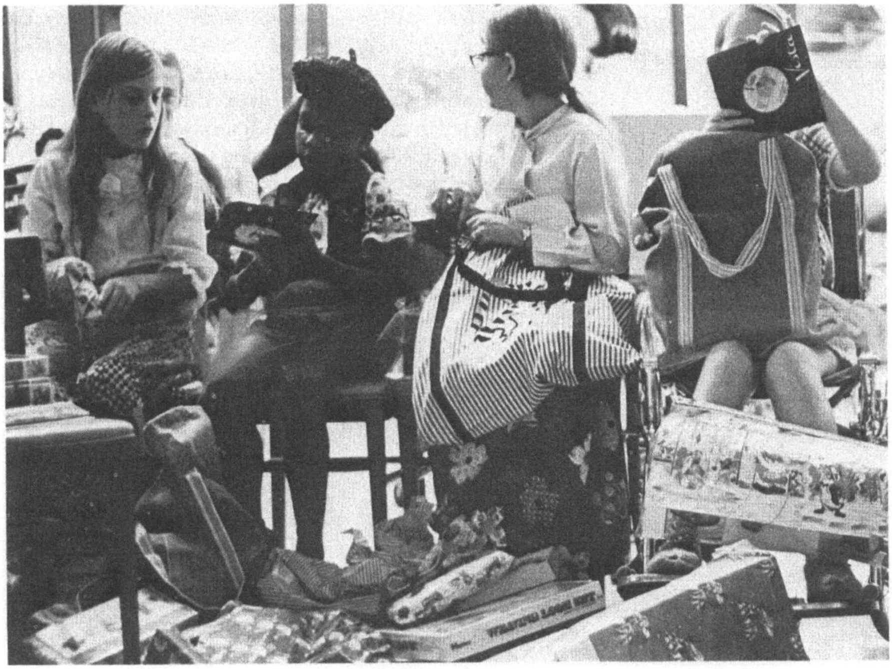

it is clearly possible to subdivide. Although an aversion for cross-sex relationships among grade school children is no longer considered axiomatic, like-sex activities predominate.[18] In addition to providing the option for girls and boys to separate, the ability to divide the multipurpose room into two or more subareas increases the possibility of a variety of simultaneous activities. One group might be constructing models and engaging in lengthy discussions over them, while another group does homework, practices a play, receives a first-aid lesson from a nurse, or engages in any number of other activities that require some level of isolation. Parents often help grade school children with their projects as well: one group might be receiving help in model building or another skill from a visiting parent.

Projects common to grade school children are preparing bag lunches for eating outdoors and making cookies or other snacks. These activities in the hospital provide several special advantages. Finicky eaters are encouraged to eat well if they have participated in the preparation of their food. Children receive basic instruction in cooking and nutrition from the hospital staff, which is particularly important for children with special dietary needs. Cooking is an enjoyable activity to engage in with visiting parents, as a snack can be an event in the hospital day.

## *Design Guidelines*

Make the multipurpose space for grade school children large enough for projects and dining to coexist. An essential characteristic of a good project space is the ability to spread out the materials and continue work throughout the day and from day to day. If the multipurpose space is large enough, several small tables beyond the number needed for everyday meal service can be available for crafts projects, board games, and other projects of considerable duration.

Design the grade school multipurpose space so that it can be easily divided into at least two separate areas. A central area surrounded by several alcoves is a good arrangement.

Provide generous closet space for the storage of materials in the multipurpose space. For craft projects, games, studying, and other activities make available a variety of art materials, tools, books, and games. Most materials can be handled readily by the children from a self-service storage area.

Provide a kitchenette in the grade school multipurpose space.

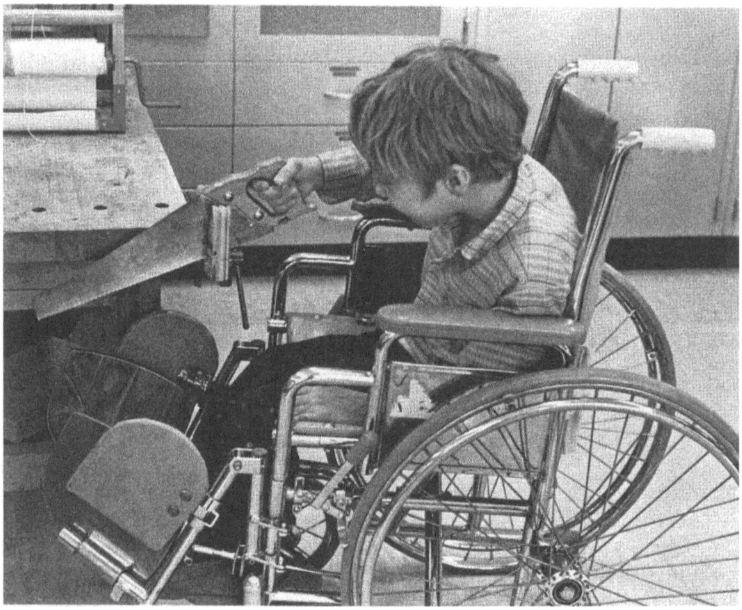

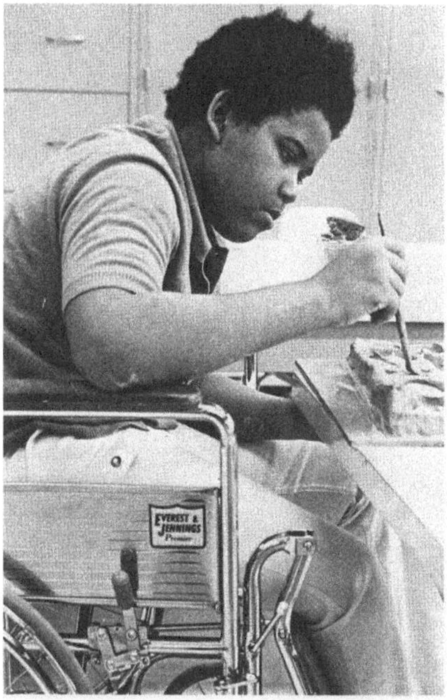
EVEREST & JENNINGS
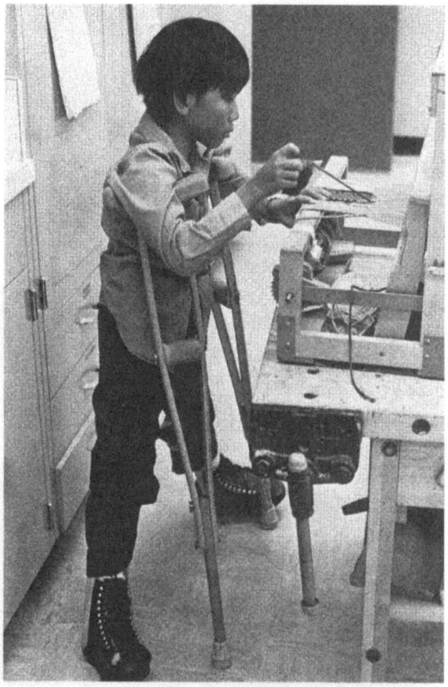
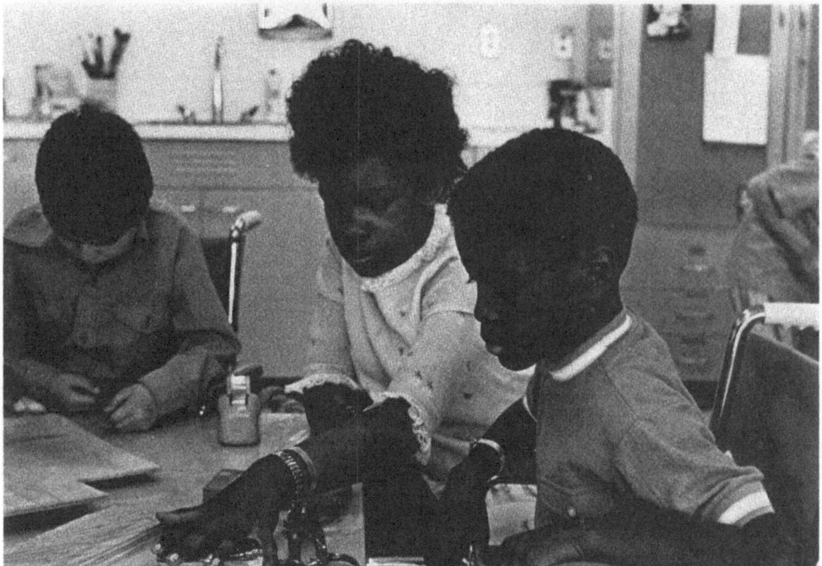

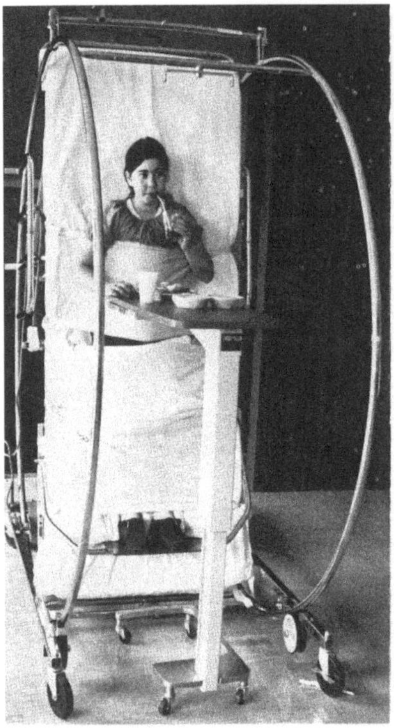

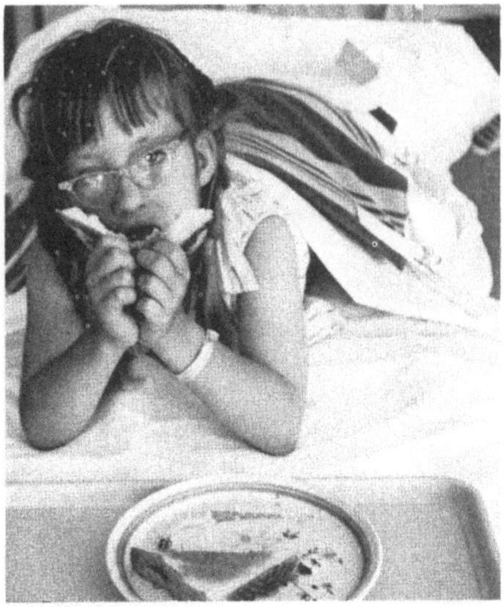

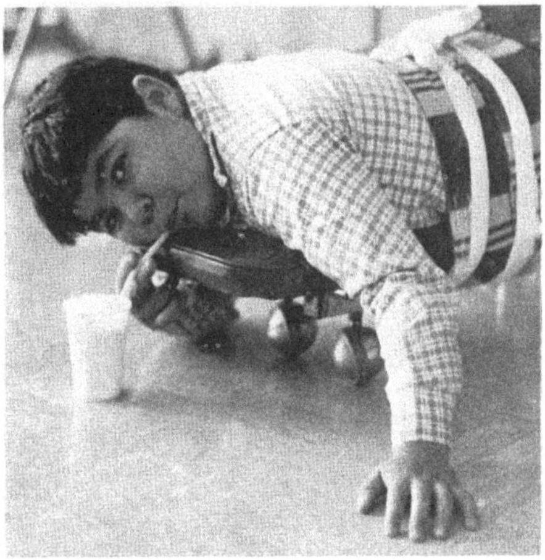

## Provide Opportunities To Assume Responsibility

During the grade school years a child normally assumes responsibility for much of his own care and for various tasks around the house that are helpful to the family. Although a child may complain about brushing his teeth, drying the dishes, or taking out the garbage, these are important steps toward accepting larger responsibilities. A sick or handicapped child who does not have these responsibilities may rightly feel unimportant and useless.

### SELF-CARE AND CARE OF PERSONAL THINGS

Wherever possible, a hospital patient should be encouraged to care for himself. For many chronically ill children, self-care will involve learning special techniques gradually over the grade school years. Although parents and nursing staff may be tempted to help out more than necessary and to keep the child in a dependent position, such action can have a major and negative effect on the child's attitude.[19]

*Design Guidelines*

Equip toilets with grab bars and other special devices necessary for the toileting of disabled or weakened children.

Provide adequate storage space for clothing, belongings, and projects in the bed area so that children can be responsible for keeping their own things in order.

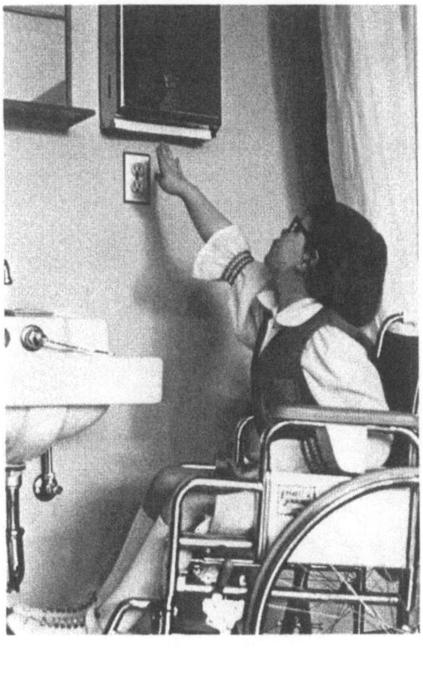

CARE OF PLANTS AND ANIMALS

For a sick child who requires constant nursing care, the ability to lavish affection and care on a pet may be essential therapy, a chance to forget oneself and to maintain a normal give-and-take existence. Unfortunately, the presence of animals in the hospital can present serious medical problems. Most animals either cause allergic reactions or carry human diseases. The expense and trouble of giving animals daily bacterial tests can be an obstacle. Many hospitals find the only practical pets to be fish, which hardly provide the warm companionship of a dog or cat.

Plants too are an important part of the grade schooler's world. He enjoys growing them, and he is curious about their growth and development. As many plants are allergenic, care must be taken in specifying plants that can be used by all the children.

*Design Guidelines*

Allow children to have nonallergenic animals. Fish and desert animals are nonallergenic and most do not carry human disease.

Provide a nonallergenic plant library so that a child can check out a live plant to put near his bed. Especially for immobilized or isolated children, living things, such as fast-growing plants, can be interesting to feed and watch. Non-allergenic plants, such as cactus and other desert plants, should be available for respiratory or allergic patients.

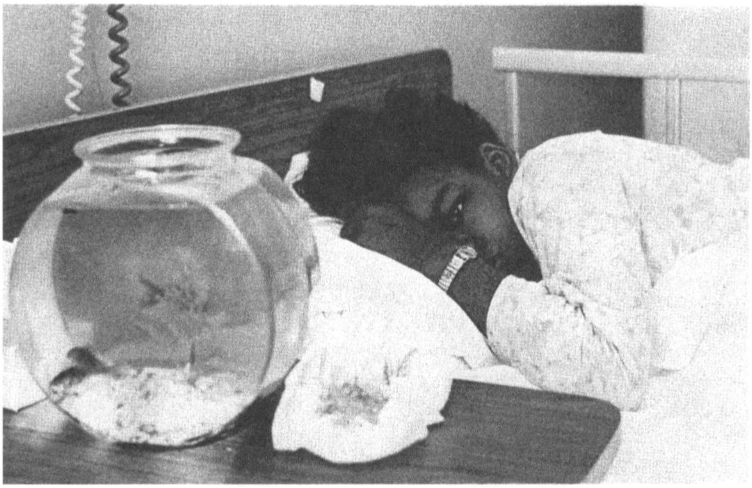

CARE OF YOUNGER CHILDREN

Grade school children often get enjoyment, entertainment, and satisfaction from caring for younger children for short periods. "The support children give each other works in both directions: older children can function as protectors or playmates for younger ones, while the helplessness of the very young, and the delight in seeing developmental changes in an infant or toddler, can act as a morale-builder for children slightly older and up to adolescence." [20]

## *Design Guidelines*

Locate the grade school nursing unit adjacent to the unit for young children so that grade school children can help in the playroom.

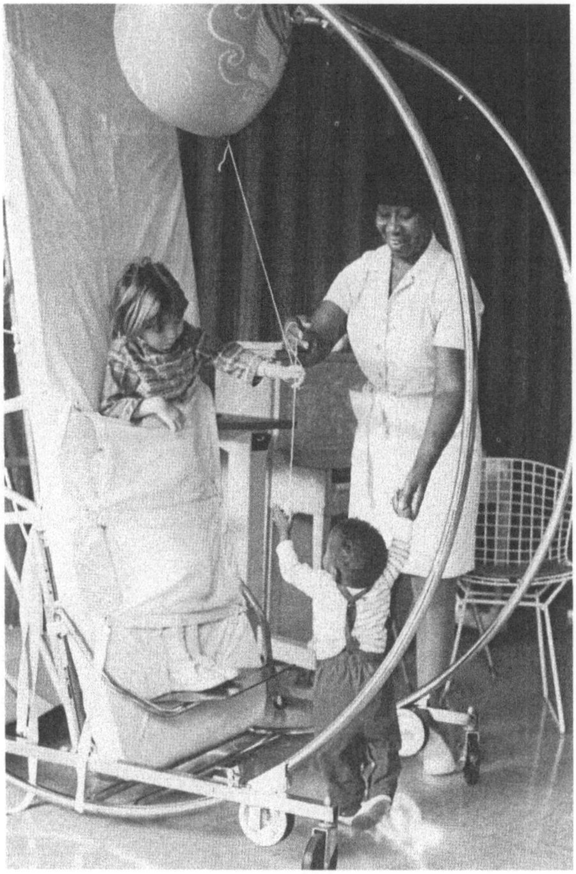

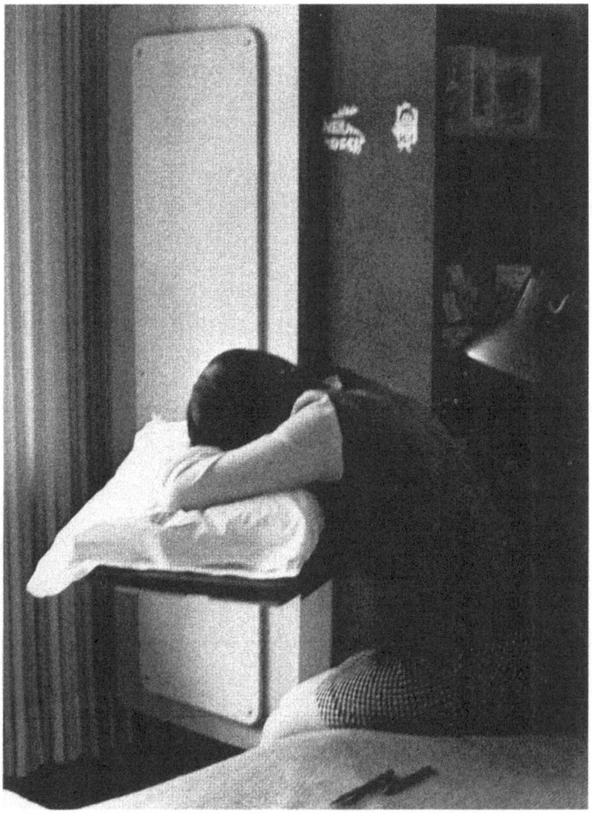

# Adolescents 6

Adolescence (12–18 years), the transitional step from childhood to adulthood, is a specific growth period characterized by a surge in biological, psychological, and social development.[1] A physical growth spurt and the appearance of secondary sexual characteristics mark the physiological level of change. In the psychological sphere, the rate of cognitive function approaches its peak, and the testing of a child's personality against the demands of the maturing psyche results in a reformulation. The exploration of value systems, personal standards, occupational and societal roles, and status as an independent but not alienated individual characterizes the social level of development.[2] Thus, the adolescent faces the task of becoming his adult self and establishing how he will relate to parents, peers, the opposite sex, school, jobs, politics, war — in short, the world.

This century's trend toward an ever earlier biological puberty, coupled with a trend toward later social and economic independence, has significantly widened the already uncomfortable gap between childhood and adulthood.[3] Although the adolescent himself is acutely, often painfully aware of his status as a member of an identifiable group, many institutions have not recognized, indeed have denied his existence and special needs. Hospitals are no exception. Despite the fact that close to half of the United States population is under the age of twenty-five, with almost forty million young people between ten and nineteen, and despite a predicted increase in the adolescent population of five percent in the next five years, medical practice and medical facilities have been slow to gear up to the problems and requirements unique to this age group.[4]

In the United States at present, youth between ten and nineteen years account for nearly ten percent of all hospital admissions.[5] Unlike younger children, these patients present medicine with illnesses more like those seen in the adult age range. They are sicker, have more medical complications, and remain in the hospital longer than do younger children Fewer of them can be expected to get completely well.[6]

## Meet Special Needs

A person in this age group is not quite an adult, yet able to assume many responsibilities. But until recent years, the adolescent "has been a medical misfit. Too old for the pediatrician and ill at ease with his parents' physician, he has had no doctor of his own. Today, at last, medicine is closing in on this long-neglected generation gap. The adolescent is recognized as a person with special health problems and with common ills complicated by anxieties that demand special understanding." [7]

As the practice of teenage medicine has grown into a subspecialty, hospitals across the country have begun to establish departments devoted exclusively to teenagers. The number and range of accommodations vary with the size of the unit, the nature of the hospital, and the average length of stay of the patient, but generally they include a variety of activity areas specifically intended for adolescent group use.[8] The University of Colorado Hospital has an eighteen-bed ward for adolescents. Children's Hospital in Los Angeles has a larger facility, thirty-two beds, for twelve-to-eighteen-year-olds. Children's Hospital in Columbus has a twenty-eight-bed teen unit. Children's Hospital at Stanford in Palo Alto contains a teen unit and includes a teen room, a day room, school facilities, and the use of a hospital recreation room with a pool table. Montefiore Hospital and Medical Center in the Bronx, New York, is planning a twenty-bed adolescent unit. Provision will be made for daily classes conducted by the Board of Education in a large room, which after school will be converted into a recreation lounge complete with ping-pong table and juke box.

In each of these hospitals special efforts have been made to help students keep up with their studies as well as providing recreational programs to occupy their time. Nonetheless, being confined to a hospital is particularly difficult for the adolescent, who fears that his illness will mar his physical appearance, compromise his body functions, and threaten his relations with the opposite sex. He resists curbs on his physical activity and is concerned about his future ability to participate in sports and to perfect athletic skills. For some adolescents the interruption from school is disastrous; others dread the social isolation from a gang or peer group. Physicians experienced in adolescent care are aware that "in adolescents, more than in any other age group, a doctor must treat the whole patient and not just his current illness." [9]

To help a teenager cope with the constraints of hospital confinement, the modern hospital should make available a variety of special facilities. These should include a place away from the bed for dining, watching TV, and studying, a quiet room where he can be alone or have a personal conversation, and a teenage sanctuary removed from hospital authority. Access to the hospital cafeteria, to recreation rooms with ping pong and pool tables, and to outdoor areas helps provide additional activities and relieve boredom, a problem common to hospitalized adolescents.[10]

If fewer than eight adolescents are grouped together, it is difficult to

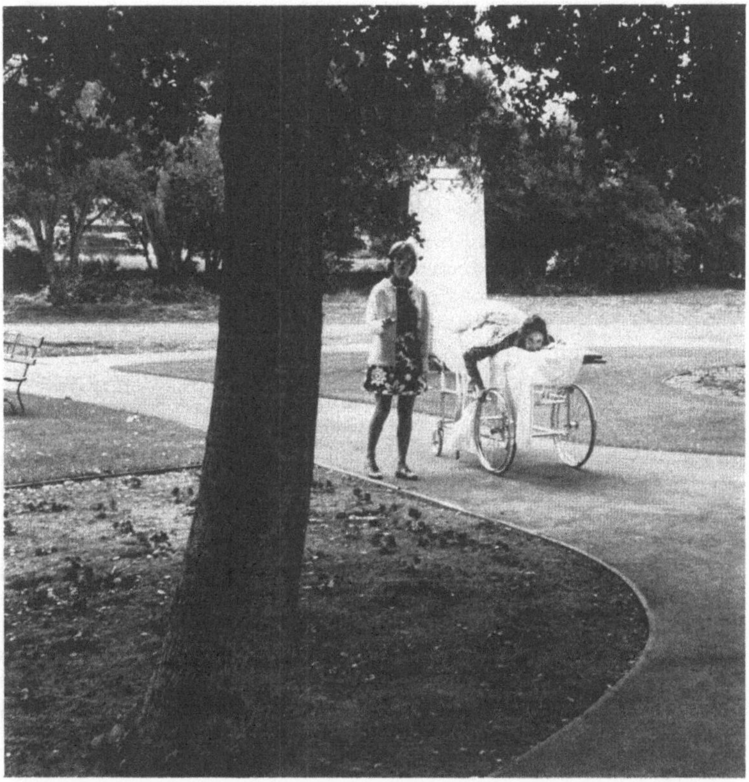

provide the special facilities required to accommodate the adolescent life style. If there are only a few adolescent patients, they will of necessity be required to share social space with other patients. A single multipurpose day room shared with younger children on the one hand, or with adults on the other, invites major conflicts. A suitable environment for young children in no way meets teenage needs. In like manner, the teenager's pattern of life, the noise he makes, and his looks and conversations can be upsetting to adult patients.[11] If more than twenty-four adolescents are confined in one area, their sheer numbers can severely tax staff ability to maintain discipline. Disruptive and challenging behavior, if beyond staff control, can handicap the operation of the unit and discourage the development of such facilities elsewhere.[12]

## *Design Guidelines*

Design units for not less than eight nor more than twenty-four patients.

## Develop a Sense of Identity

As he matures, the adolescent gradually develops concepts of his own identity, both as an individual and as a member of a group. Hospitalization, however, poses a very real threat to the newly developing sense of identity and independence of the adolescent, who may attempt to safeguard these achievements by resisting authority.[13] The adolescent occasionally needs respite from the hospital staff and routine in order to cope with and overcome these concerns.[14] The hospital can assist him in maintaining his developmental gains by providing appropriate places of retreat, such as a teen sanctuary, a teen day-room, and a quiet room.

The concept of "personal space" or "personal territory" has been well described by students of animal behavior, and it has been studied more recently by anthropologists, social psychologists, and a few architects.[15] The size and impersonal nature of the hospital make the need for a personal space there overwhelming. The need obviously increases with the length of stay, but even with short periods of hospitalization, patients try to personalize their space with the display of "get-well" cards, snapshots, and posters, although personal decoration is generally discouraged in the hospital. The rules that make room decoration difficult, while motivated in part by the desire of the staff to maintain an ascetic and clean front, are also dictated by obsolete theories of contagion. Hospital rooms must be designed so that patients can make nonpermanent changes. One approach is to provide magnetic surfaces on which to mount posters and decorations. Another is to provide a way of hanging things from the ceiling. The very real problems of maintenance, cleanliness, and asepsis require innovative solutions, but unless the need is recognized, the barren environment will continue.

#### BEDROOM

The hospital bedroom is a multipurpose environment, where the patient sleeps, is examined and treated, studies, visits, dresses, performs toilet functions, bathes, and often eats. When occupied by more than one person, the hospital bedroom must accommodate a range of social situations as well as the most private functions.[16] The conflicting needs for privacy and community within the single space of the hospital bedroom make it one of the more difficult design problems. It is particularly important to resolve the conflict in use for teenage occupants because of their particular sensitivity to body, sex, appearance, and infirmities, coupled with the need for social intercourse.[17]

The rationale for the current trend toward private bedrooms found in several new teenage units may be based partially on the experience and desires of teenagers in college dormitories, where an individual room is ranked high. In fact, the hospitalized teenager has a very different set of problems from the student in the dormitory. A student has freedom of choice. If he doesn't like his roommate, he can move to another room.

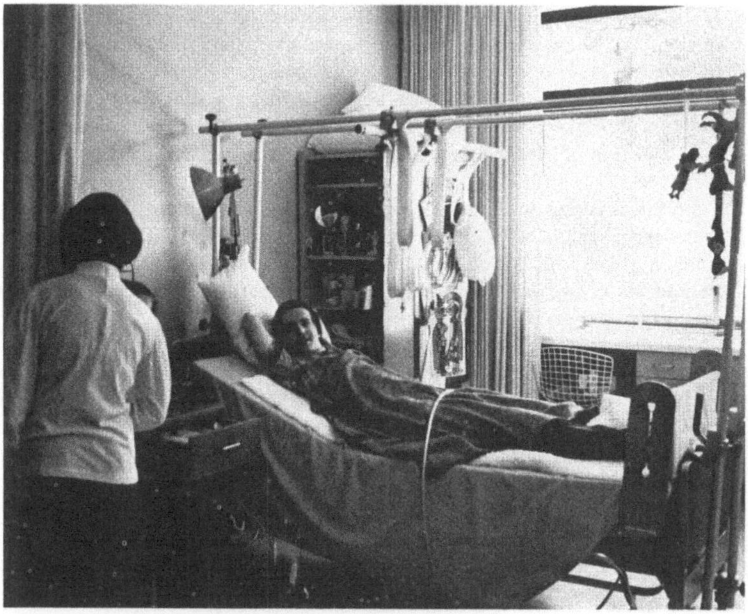

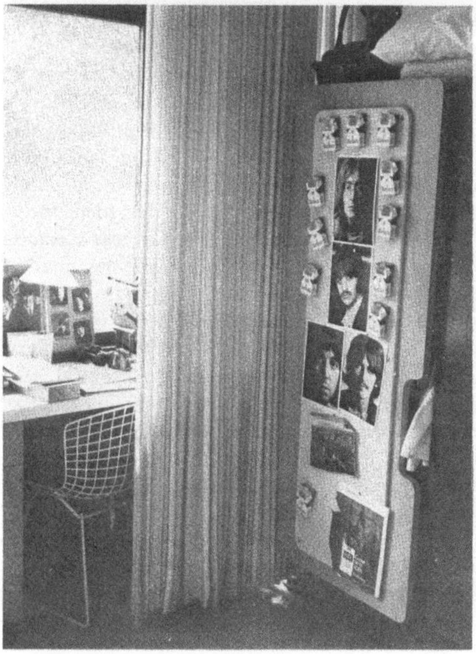

If he is lonely, he can seek friends outside of his private room. The hospitalized teenager has no such options, particularly if he is confined to bed. It is a vexing problem simultaneously to meet the hospitalized teenager's needs for community space to foster social relationships and for personal space to support his privacy. The ideal solution would provide a choice of either privacy or community as desired by the individual teenager.

Four-bed rooms provide the opportunity for company, conversation, and friendship, which helps prevent depression and withdrawal. At the same time, a patient in a four-bed room has relatively more privacy than a patient in a two-bed room, for he can withdraw from the group with greater ease than if he had a single roommate.

The disadvantages of a four-bed room center around its lack of absolute privacy, whether for personal body functions, for intimate conversations, and for pursuing individual habits of sleeping and reading without disturbing other patients. Generally, a curtain suspended from a ceiling curtain track surrounds the hospital beds and serves to separate patients from each other. This is a highly unsatisfactory form of separation. Bathroom noise and conversation are easily overheard. The odor of toileting invades the rest of the room, to the discomfort and embarrassment of all patients. An indiscreet person may whisk open the curtain and expose an undressed, sensitive teenager to public view.

Conflicting habits of the diverse individuals in the multibed room result in a second set of problems. Teenagers have erratic hours: some like to read late at night, others watch television, still others converse. The teenager likes to be able to carry out these activities in bed rather than in another area. Audio privacy for TV and radio can be easily accommodated by earphones, but the disturbance caused by reading lights or TV pictures produces a problem as yet unsolved. Visiting families and friends, particularly those of the opposite sex, add even more conflict. There is no privacy for conversation. A quiet room designed for this purpose can be used only if the patient is ambulatory or has transportation.

A double room offers the opportunity to develop a more personal relationship with one's roommate than is generally possible in a four-bed room. Such interaction can be particularly supportive if the other person has a similar medical problem. For example, Dan, an eighteen-year-old with a long-term spinal problem who was observed in the hospital, stated that a good roommate made the hospital experience worthwhile. His roommate, Carl, was seventeen and in the hospital for the first time for a spinal operation. Dan, who had already had the operation, was able to comfort Carl with realistic information, sympathy, and humor. The double room is also valuable for persons who have trouble relating to others but who still require companionship. This asset takes on particular importance when patients have to be in the hospital over a long period of time.

Single rooms must be provided on every adolescent unit for the very sick, for some infectious patients, for dying patients, and occasionally for

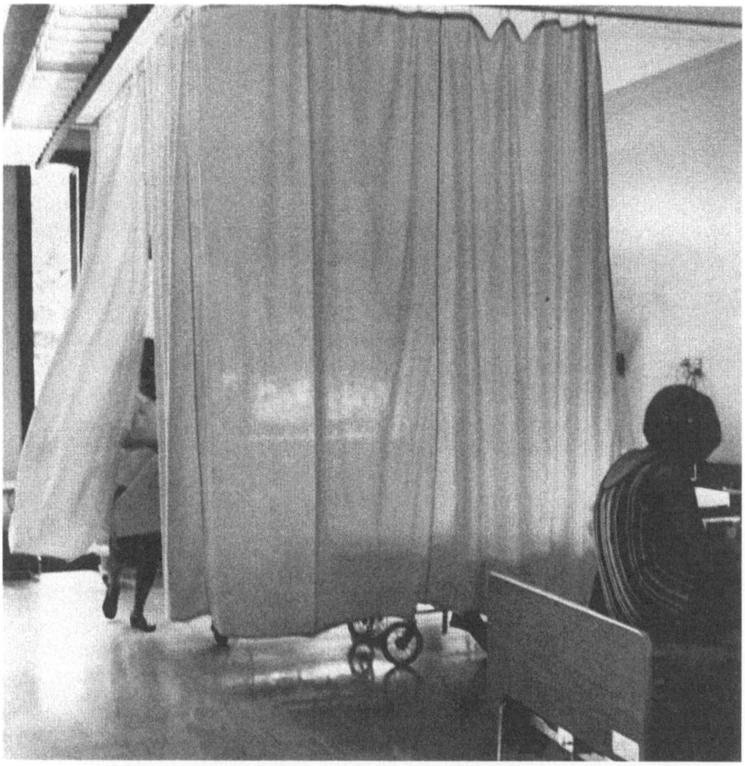

emotionally disturbed patients. These rooms should be used interchangeably, so that no one room becomes identified as the room for dying. The single rooms should be closest to the nursing station and should be visible to the nurse from her seat. The room should have its own bathroom, designed for isolation, for parents, or for other functions as they arise.

## *Design Guidelines*

Provide a variety of room accommodations, including single rooms, double rooms, and four-bed rooms.

Surround every hospital teenage bed with a space large enough to accommodate medical equipment and personal possessions.

Identify a clearly defined territory in which each teenager can keep his possessions and personalize his environment. The space needed by a teenager for his personal possessions includes both hanging space, shelf space, and drawer space.

Teenagers generally have a greater number of "necessary" objects than adults, including musical instruments, record players, radios and books, as well as hair dryers, beauty aids, and personal clothing.

Assure each patient in a multibed room olfactory, acoustical, and visual privacy while performing personal functions, reading at night, or watching TV. The creative ingenuity of the building designers must be devoted to the development of a screen or divider that a patient can operate from his bed and that will have olfactory, acoustical, and visual screening properties. Exploration should be made of the possible uses of low masking sound near a patient's bed to act as white noise and minimize specific sounds. Individual ventilation systems should be studied, as well as new night lighting devices. The problem of adequate separation between patients affects not only teenagers but all adult patients and is a crying hospital need.

Place every patient bed next to a window and in a corner of the room. If given a choice, a patient will select a bed by a window or by a corner, in that order of preference. The middle bed in a row of three is considered the least desirable. In corporate offices, the status of the executive is expressed by his relationship first to a private office, then to a window in a group space, then to his proximity to a corner. In Synanon, patients are rewarded for good behavior by being assigned sleeping space progressively nearer and nearer to the corner of a large dormitory room.

Make all bedroms able to be observed casually as one passes down the hall. The degree of openness will be affected by the location of bathrooms and other spaces off the corridor. For some rooms a half-glazed door provides adequate supervision; other rooms need a window with a movable curtain.

Hospitalization is a period of stress. The ability to cope with physical and emotional problems requires quiet in order to collect one's thoughts. Teenagers need a place to be alone, to reflect or meditate, and to engage in quiet conversation with family, doctor, nurse, or close friends.

In the hospital, chapels may serve the need for personal meditation. An outdoor secluded garden with the proper restful quality can also be used. But in addition, a "quiet room" for intimate conversations and undisturbed relaxation is essential. There is always danger that such a small, pleasant room in a hospital unit will be taken over for a thousand and one other purposes, unless the medical importance of keeping this type of space available is recognized.

## *Design Guidelines*

Plan space for a small, pleasant room on every teen unit large enough for about six people to talk in comfortably. One or two of the people may be on gurneys or in wheelchairs.

Maintain a low light level.

Make the floor soft and comfortable.

Decorate the room in mute tones, perhaps focusing on a view into a quiet garden.

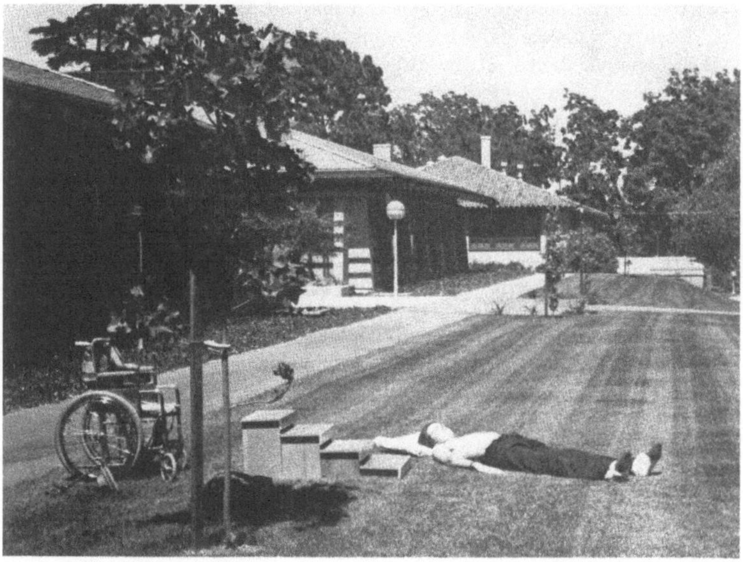

## Allow for Maintaining a Positive Body Image

Personal appearance and personal hygiene are very important to an adolescent's developing body image. He is sensitive and vulnerable about the physical aspect of his person and the rapid and major changes occurring in his body.

Many teenagers spend hours in front of the mirror. All teenagers are self-conscious about minor flaws or irregularities in their complexions or figures. Sick teenagers are particularly self-conscious about their physical appearance. Adolescents also place a great deal of importance on body modesty. Both girls and boys are highly embarrassed by the exposure of their body and bodily functions in the hospital.[18] The hospital can offer support to these needs in adolescence through sensitive arrangement of its facilities for personal care.

### BATHROOM

The image of a hospital as a sterile, unfriendly place is epitomized in the stark asepsis of hospital bathrooms. Ceramic tile and stainless steel reinforce the negative image of the "institution." Most present hospital bathrooms open directly off the bedroom. The convenience and space-saving nature of this arrangement must be weighed against the loss of privacy. Entering that silent door from a bedroom announces to everyone that "one is about to use the bathroom." When visitors are in a room, both visitors and patients are sensitive about using a bathroom opening directly off the bedroom, and patients will often refrain from using it out of sensitivity until visitors have left. More privacy is provided if there is an anteroom between a bedroom or day room and the bathroom.

Teenagers dislike gang bathrooms. In a high school girls' locker room, it is common to see all the girls queuing up for a single private shower stall while the huge gang showers stand empty.

Maintaining a pleasing appearance is one way to maintain morale. Illness often threatens personal attractiveness — a threat that is particularly frightening for a teenager who has not yet developed a great deal of self-confidence. It is important for a disabled teenager to have equipment and space available to help him keep up with normal grooming standards. In an institution such as the hospital, the bathtub room may be the only place where one can be truly alone to meditate without the possibility of disturbance. Even the hospital tub room can be an attractive, richly colored place with green growing plants, encouraging relaxation. Bathroom design in general must provide visual, olfactory, and acoustic privacy, as well as safety and convenience.

*Design Guidelines*

Avoid opening bathrooms directly off living spaces, such as bedrooms or day rooms. An intermediate space or corridor should act as a barrier between the living space and the bathroom.

Put the bathtub in a room separate from, but adjacent to, a toilet and lavatory.

Avoid gang bathrooms in hospitals. Each toilet and wash-basin should be in a room with a door that separates it from the adjacent spaces. The wash basin should be in the same room as the toilet to facilitate hand washing.

Make it possible to open doors to hospital bathtub rooms and toilets with minimum pressure. Persons in wheelchairs and on crutches may be quite capable of self-care but not strong enough to open a heavy door.

Construct bathroom doors that slide or swing out. There is real danger that if a person falls or faints in the bathroom or toilet, the door will be blocked.[19]

Make bathrooms and bathroom compartments large enough so that patients can be helped by an attendant if necessary.[20]

Make bathrooms attractive places for dressing and self-care.

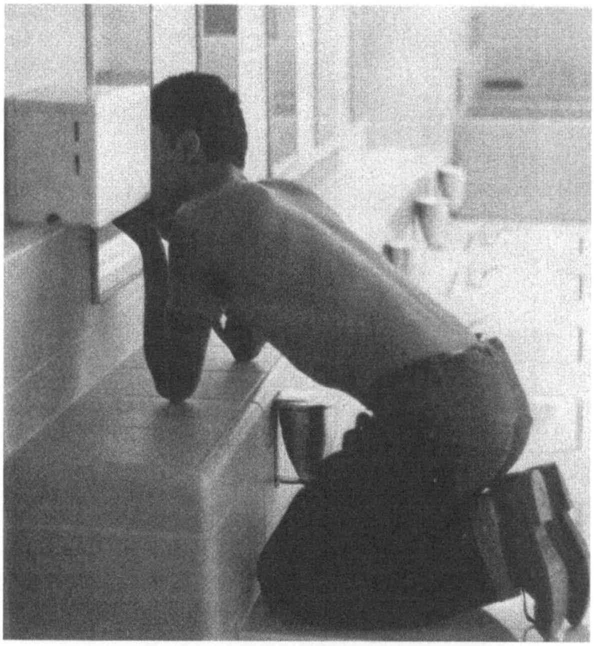

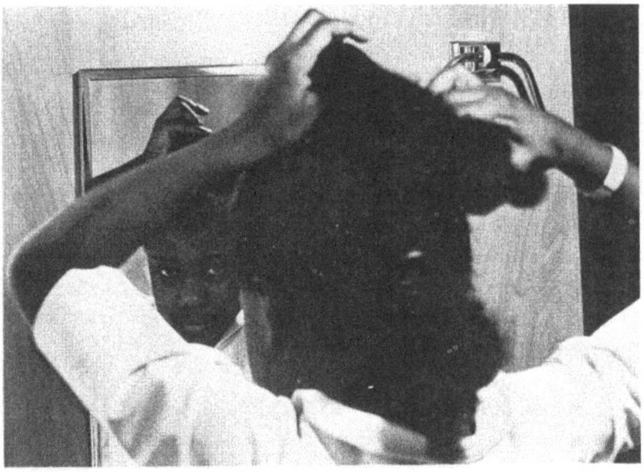

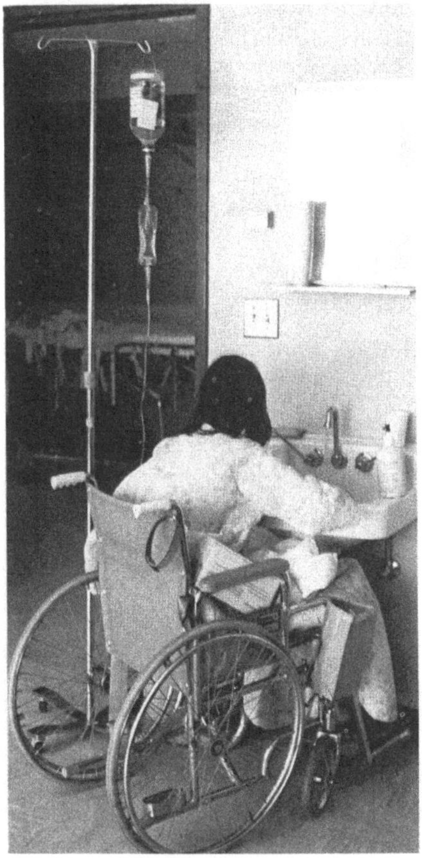

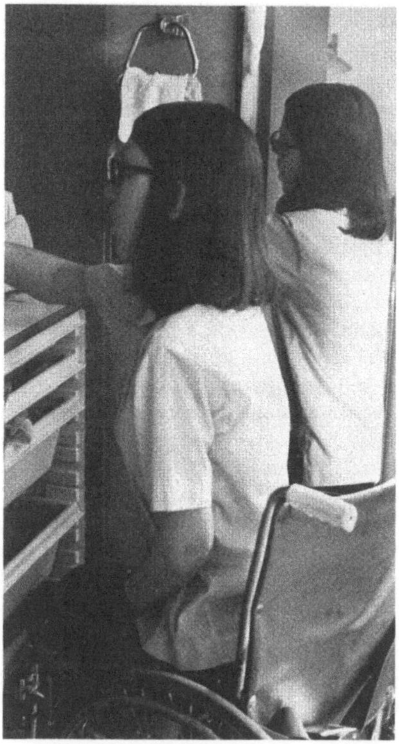

LAUNDRY FACILITIES

When teens are hospitalized for more than a few days, the question of dress becomes important. Choice of clothing communicates basic feelings to other teens. It is important to encourage this form of self-expression, even though from the hospital administration point of view it would be easier to provide standard robes and pajamas.

*Design Guidelines*

Include space for a washer, dryer, ironing board, and sewing machine on every teen unit. Teenagers usually care for their own clothes and personal belongings. Keeping one's things neat and clean boosts morale as well as providing something to do.

## Foster Individual Independence and Responsibility

Being confined to a hospital imposes more restrictions and controls than most adolescents are prepared to cope with. Just at the period in his life when the adolescent has achieved a degree of independence and is not restricted territorially to a house, a neighborhood, or perhaps even to a city, he finds himself in a hospital where activity, time, and space are structured for him.

The adolescent may express his fears and anxiety through excessive assertions of independence from routine, violence and damage to hospital property, or defiance of rules relative to school work, sex, smoking, or drugs. The hospital must recognize the adolescent's needs and fears rather than accentuating them, and must try to provide a delicate balance between security, support, and control on the one hand, and the opportunity for independence, self-expression, and freedom on the other.

Parents expect a hospital to exercise appropriate control and regulation over their children. The role of the hospital *in loco parentis* has a considerable effect on the adolescent unit administration, with the result that the hospital may not be completely free to strike a bargain between its own policies and the desires of the parents. Problems related to sex, drugs, smoking, and fighting sometimes occur where diverse groups of teenagers congregate. The frustrations of the confined and ill teenager increase the possibility of these problems.

#### TEEN SANCTUARY

Teenagers must have a place of their own in the hospital, away from adult interference, where they can be their own masters. It should be a place where they can all get together to talk with visiting friends or friends made in the hospital, to play music loudly without disturbing a sleeping roommate, and to escape from the younger patients. For this reason, adolescents need more square footage per patient than any other child or adult patients.[21]

At home, teenagers identify their own spaces. Pictures of heroes, posters, clippings, notes, and varied artwork define their particular place, even when a room is shared with several others. Teenagers often reject attractive places provided by adults, even though they themselves might not select anything very different. Part of the enjoyment of a place is being able to affect it as one chooses.

Teenagers do not like to be too open to the authority of the hospital staff. At the same time, however, the hospital is responsible for their activities. Adolescents are often quite capable of setting up and caring for their own space if given enough leeway. A satisfactory arrangement would allow the nursing staff to look in occasionally as they pass the sanctuary door. Teenagers will not use a room that is under constant adult surveillance.

Music is a symbol of teen culture. Teenagers like to fill the space around them with music at loud volume. Popular sounds and musicians change rapidly, and young people need to keep in touch with these tastes while

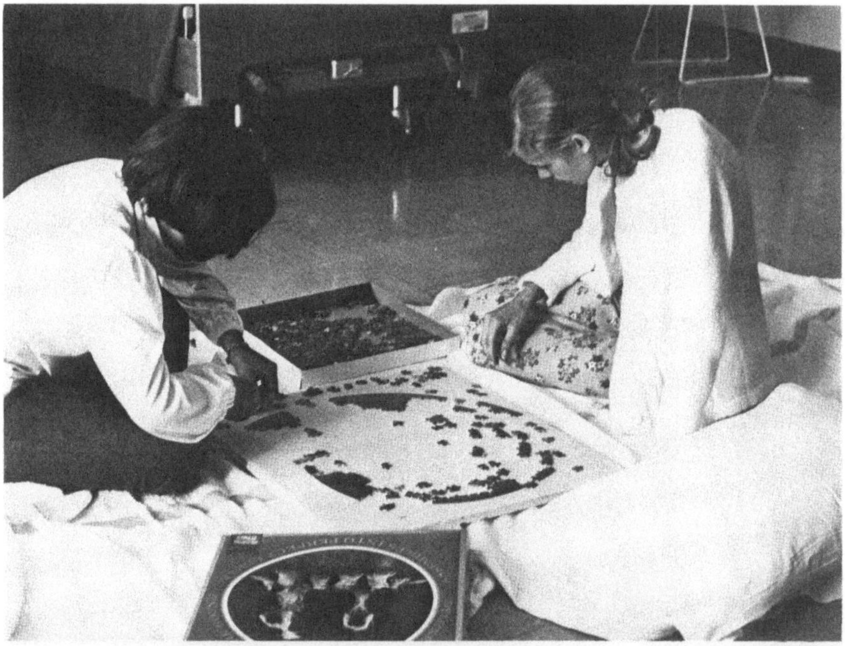

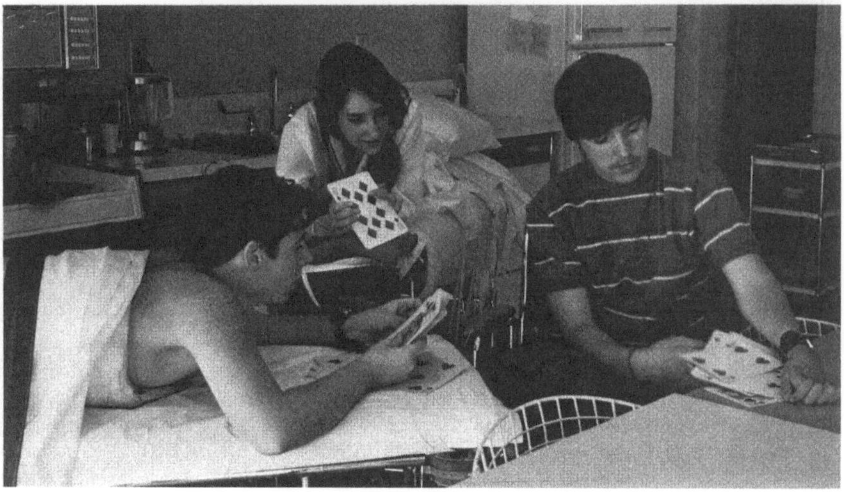

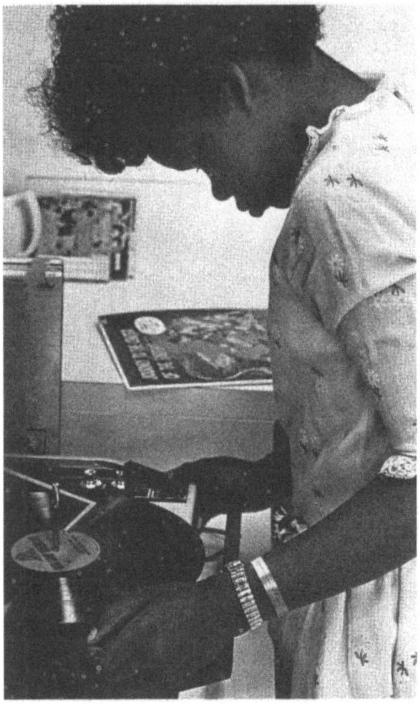

in the hospital and to share them with others. Music can also be an important emotional outlet for a musician. Many teenagers play instruments and in so doing find release from feelings of depression, fear, and loneliness. Music also encourages dance and offers a chance to be boisterous, to let off steam. At home or at popular concerts teenagers sit around on the floor or share large pillows. Chairs, like conservative clothing, belong to adult culture.

The availability of food in a teen room is an excellent reason for dropping in to see what is happening, as well as for lingering if something interesting is going on. It has been reported that eating is "the one common activity that ostensibly brings people together to fulfill individual desires, but often allows people the 'opening' for communal activities. Some restaurants and most coffee houses are places where this happens. The kitchen during a party at home is often the most used space for discussions. Somehow it's easier for people to get together over passing each other food than simply introducing themselves." [22]

It is uncomfortable to talk with someone whose eyes are on a very different level. Looking up and looking down have hierarchal connotations not conducive to free exchange. Teenagers must be on an eye level with one another, whether they arrive by a gurney, a bed, in a wheelchair, or on foot.

*Design Guidelines*

Make the room large enough for use by a small group of teenagers. A room larger than 400 square feet is no longer homey and appears empty and uninviting when used by only a few people. A smaller room does not provide enough space for dancing and cannot accommodate a group of friends or several gurneys.

Include a snack bar in the teen sanctuary. A modest hot plate and soft drink arrangement is enough, for more elaborate facilities would involve clean-up problems.

Make the floor comfortable for sitting.

Free the teen sanctuary of close visual supervision.

Isolate the teen sanctuary acoustically from the rest of the hospital and provide a phonograph and an AM-FM radio.

Make furniture, decorations, and lighting changeable. Each new group of teenagers must be able to arrange its own space.

## Develop Peer Group Relations

Adolescence is a period when friends of both sexes are important. Adolescents study in groups, work on joint projects, eat together, play music and dance together, talk together endlessly in person and on the telephone, and watch television together with friends or family. An adolescent feels lost and isolated in the hospital where his friends may not be able to visit.

### TEEN DAY ROOM

A teen day room is a place where teenagers, nurses, doctors, family, and friends can come together. It is territory common to both adolescents and adults. At home, eating, studying, and TV watching take place in a living-dining area or kitchen. Studying is sometimes accomplished with the television set on. The hospital must provide a similar multiuse group facility.

The entire teen unit should be able to gather together in the day room to talk, play, or eat, although sometimes some patients will dine elsewhere, and some visitors will eat with the patients. The activities in the day room require different light intensities. Eating is more pleasant if the level of lighting is low, whereas studying and close work require bright illumination.

*Design Guidelines*

Make the room large enough to accommodate up to twenty people, some of whom will be on gurneys, in wheelchairs, or in beds.

Arrange food service at several small tables, each seating four persons, which can be grouped together for different eating arrangements.

Allow for varying the level of the lighting, depending on the nature of the activity taking place.

Construct at least two alcoves off the general day room area. An area off the central space will allow patients to work on projects without having to remove them when meals are being served. An alcove will also allow a person to watch what is going on from a secure vantage point without having to participate in the activity: "Studies of seating pat-

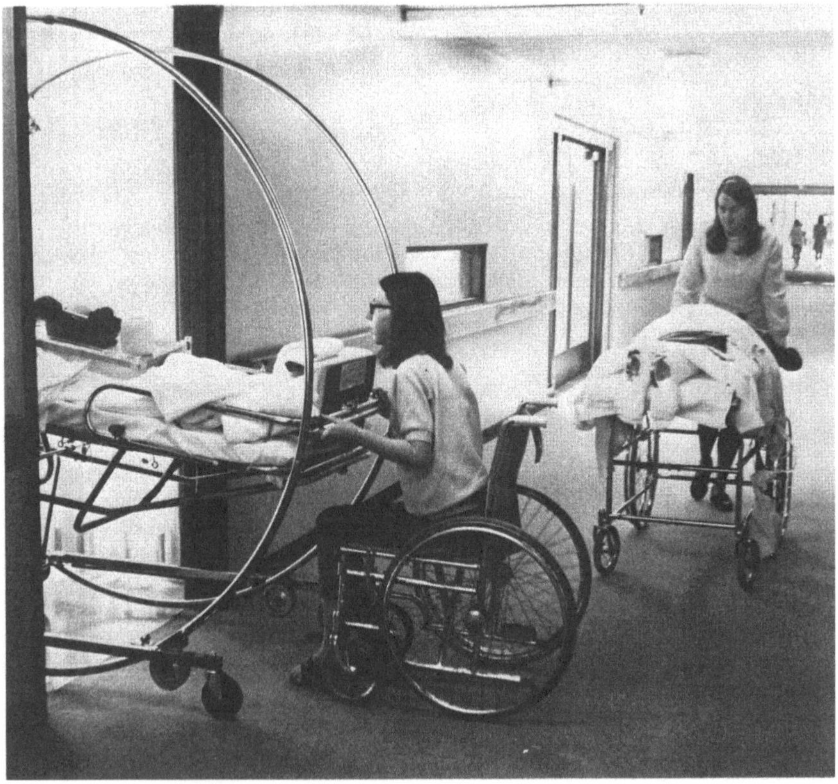

terns of groups of people, both healthy individuals and patients of various sorts . . . showed that people like to sit with their backs to walls and other tangible barriers. Part of this is simply because of comfort and the possibility of leaning one's chair back against a solid surface, but there also seems to be a need for security." [23]

Design a kitchenette adjacent to the day room. Teenagers snack continuously, especially when studying and at bedtime. They also enjoy occasional cooking and might like to prepare food for use in the teen sanctuary. If the hospital were to relax the morning routine, a teenager might welcome the opportunity to sleep late and prepare his own breakfast. Teenagers on special diets can assume the responsibility for choosing their own foods correctly with the guidance of staff.

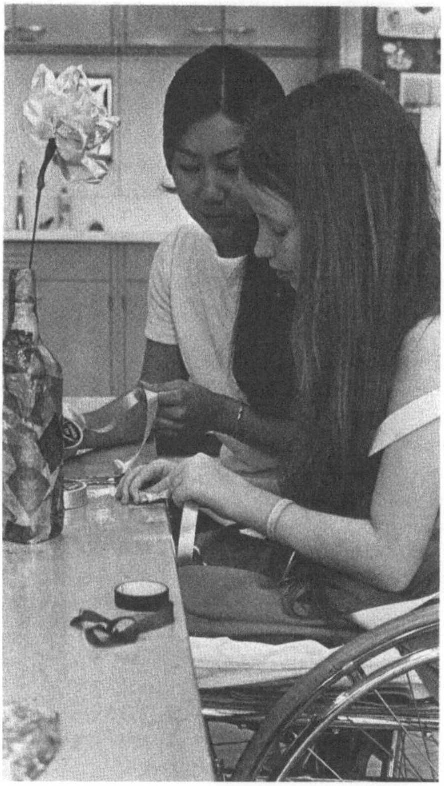

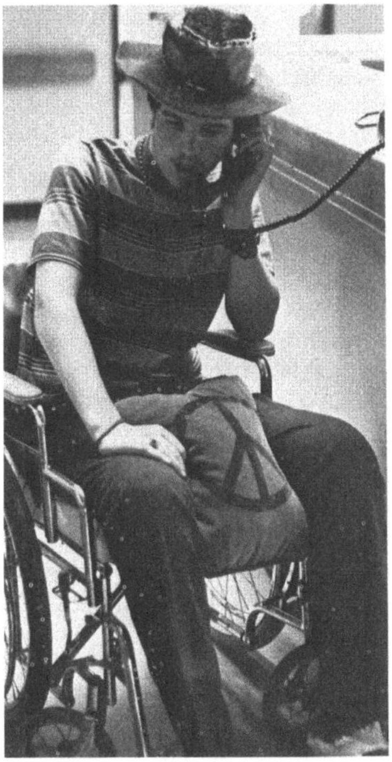

TELEPHONES

The telephone is an accepted and necessary phenomenon in the life of the modern teenager. In the hospital, the phone as a means of communication takes on special significance because it may be the only source of contact with friends. In times of stress, conversation about highly confidential worries and hopes assume great importance. A teenager's confidant may be another teenager with whom contact is possible only by telephone. There is not sufficient privacy in a shared bedroom to conduct intimate conversations. Provisions must be made for private telephoning for wheelchair and gurney patients. Besides the obvious need for personal communication with friends, the telephone has potential as an important education tool, as further developments in electronic learning systems appear.

## *Design Guidelines*

Provide a telephone jack by every hospital bed.

Include an enclosed telephone alcove large enough to accommodate a wheelchair or gurney patient.

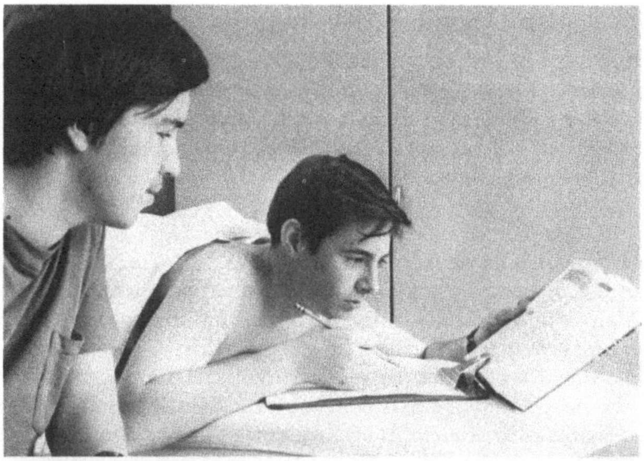

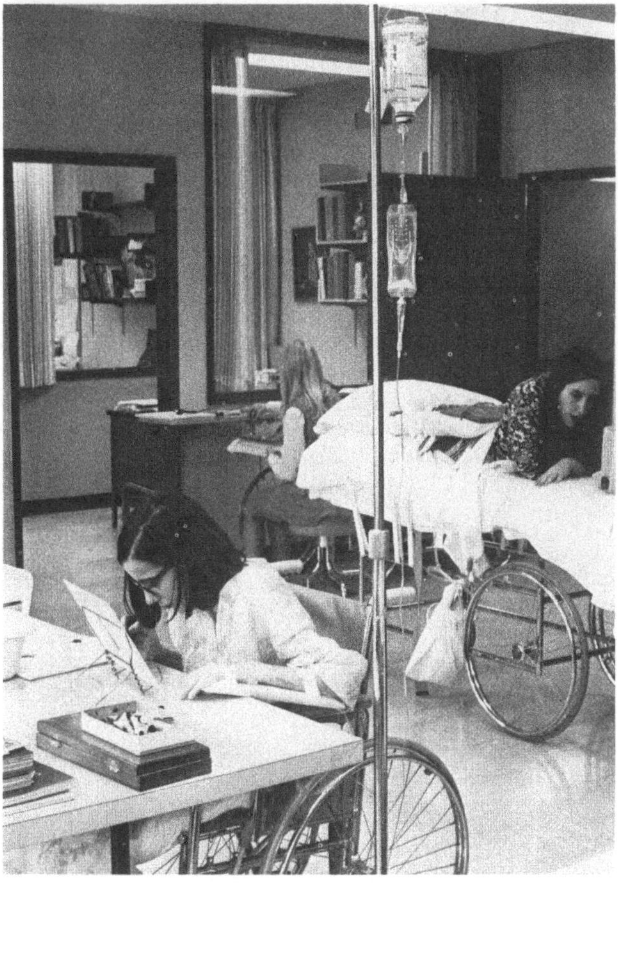

## Provide for Cognitive Development

Adolescence brings with it an upsurge in the rate of intellectual development. For the young person who is studying in preparation for a job or college, illness and hospitalization are seriously disrupting. For the teenager with school problems, absence owing to hospitalization makes a bad situation worse.

The hospital must make every effort to support continuity of schooling for its adolescent patients, especially those who stay for long periods. Facilities such as schoolrooms, desk space in the bedrooms, and electronic learning devices aid the teenager in keeping up with his schoolwork.

Many school systems provide both books and teachers for patients in the hospital to enable them to stay abreast of schoolwork. Additional audio-visual tools, such as tapes, slides, and movies, are now available. In the near future, special communication links in some universities will also enable each student in his own dormitory room to dial the university's central library of audio-visual material or to connect with the university's computer. The university systems may thus be fully integrated with the public network, giving schools throughout the city, and individual students in their homes or community centers, immediate access to the resources of the university. Educational programs can be arranged through local colleges. Lectures or even term-length courses can be made available. The pediatric unit of a hospital, particularly the teenage center, is a natural location for this type of service.

### *Design Guidelines*

Provide a hospital schoolroom for adolescents.

Equip a room with appropriate audio-visual and electronic learning equipment, designed to accommodate a patient prone, seated, or standing.

Provide every bed with a phone jack to be used as a communication link.

# Family Participation 7

When a child is hospitalized, both the family and the child face numerous fears, problems, and stresses. Children in hospitals suffer not only because they are sick but also because they are uprooted from their own environments at a point in their development when they depend most on the care and security of family life. Only recently has medicine begun to focus on the importance of the family to the child's welfare and the effect on the family group of the illness and hospitalization of one of its members.[1]

In the past decade, leading British authorities in the field of child care have singled out the ability of one or both parents to be with the young child as the factor of greatest significance in helping both parents and child to cope successfully with the trauma of hospitalization.[2] From these and other studies on the reactions of children and families to a child's illness and hospitalization, it has been found that many children experience harmful effects simply from being in the hospital, quite aside from their specific illnesses. This suffering takes on different forms and degrees of severity depending on the age level of the child, the length of separation from the family, the seriousness and pain of the illness, and the background of both parent and child.[3] Moreover, the suffering is compounded if the child speaks a different language from the staff, or if the child feels unwanted, as in the case of the black child in a segregated hospital or in a hospital where the staff comes from a different ethnic, cultural, and economic background.

Parents can often shield their children from their most flagrant fears, both real and imaginary, yet most hospitals effectively discourage parent participation, both through their policies and through the reflection of those policies in the hospital's physical design. At one time the stated reasons for keeping parents away from their children were to prevent contagion and the spread of infectious disease and to maintain discipline and quiet. In 1907, for example, it was observed that "one source of care and annoyance of officials in children's hospitals comes from the fact that mothers are so often determined to remain with their sick children . . . The mother should never be allowed to remain in the ward and thus demoralize the discipline of the hospital and the other children." [4] With the advent of antibiotics and the shift in disease patterns away from a major emphasis on contagious diseases toward an emphasis on congenital disorders, the reasons for isolating children from their parents have lost validity. Despite the change in need, however, the old forms persist, and today, although many hospitals have unlimited visiting hours for parents, only a few allow parents to stay overnight or to participate in the care of the child.[5]

Even in cases where parent involvement has been encouraged, fathers have often felt out of place. Arthur Colman notes the disparity between his impressions of husbands in the maternity hospital setting, where they appeared "weak and ineffectual," and in their own homes, where they were relaxed and confident.[6] Nursing is traditionally a feminine occupation. The role of comforting, feeding, tidying up, and bathing the child has been characterized as "woman's work." The feminine atmosphere discourages many fathers who might want to help care for a sick child and thus deprives the child of his father's presence.

The case for parent participation in the care of the hospitalized child is predicated on a healthy relationship between parent and child, on the parent being free of more pressing responsibilities at home or at work, and on the parent having some faith in the hospital and the staff. There are times when parents cannot or should not spend much time in the hospital with their children, as when they need the opportunity of the child's absence in the hospital to obtain a desperately needed respite, particularly if the child has been ill at home for a prolonged period. Other parents do not want to be with their children in the hospital.[7] Some even upset their children, so that it is better for both the child and the parents if they do not stay. A parent who fears and distrusts the hospital can transfer his fears to the child, although usually a parent's presence with a child provides a supportive function.

But parents with children in hospitals are themselves worried, concerned, and uprooted from their daily routine. They too need an atmosphere of empathy and understanding. They should be made to feel that they belong with their hospitalized child, that their presence is welcomed by the hospital staff. Community workers serving as hospital hosts can help, perhaps better than any others, in making a parent feel wanted and comfortable. The hospital can also effectively demonstrate a willingness for parent participation by providing the facilities required to make parents' visits to sick children as comfortable, pleasant, and easy as possible.

Levels of family participation range from that of a parent providing total care for his child as in Care-by-Parent units to that of a parent visiting for a brief period of time. Each condition requires its own set of physical facilities. The hospital environment should provide the range of accommodations necessary for different levels of participation by *both* parents and should minimize the difficulties for families in various situations.

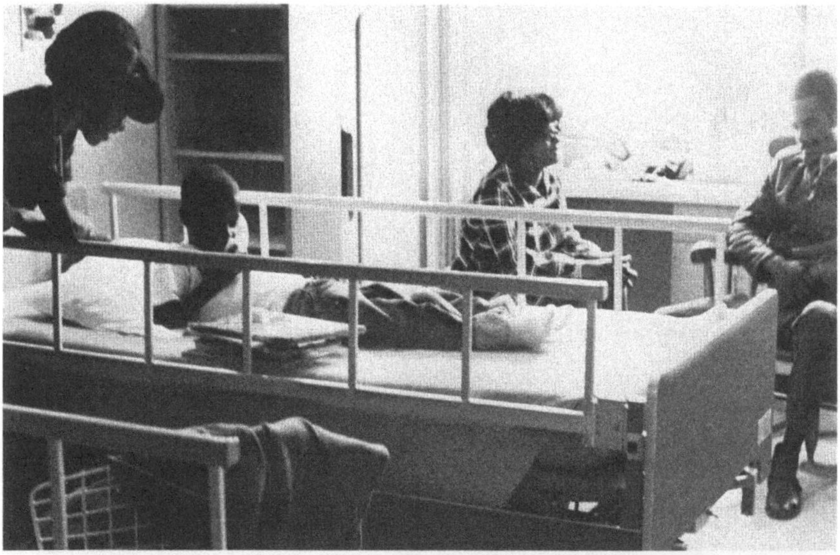

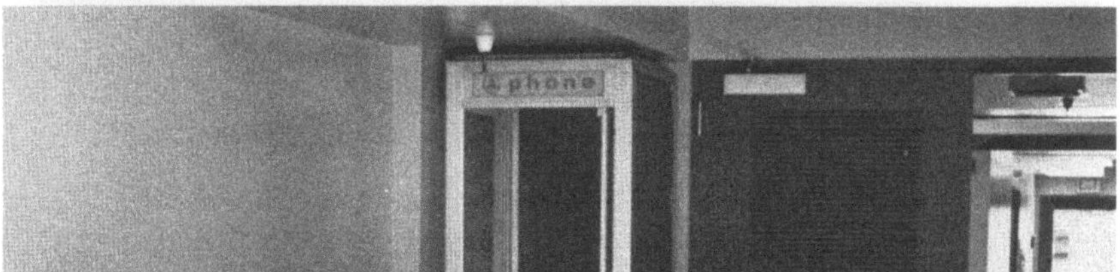
phone

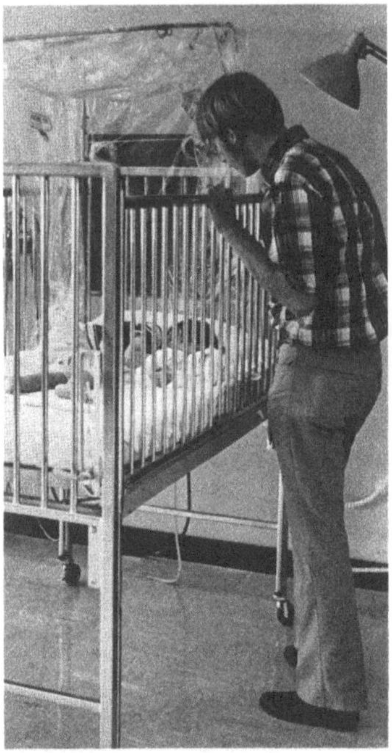

## Provide Outside Facilities and Services To Enable Parents To Be with Their Children When Needed

More and more hospitals are becoming centers of regional specialties in medicine. The families of patients who come from outlying areas therefore require inexpensive accommodations. Yet health insurance plans do not cover hotel and restaurant expenses. Because families with ill children generally experience financial stress as well, they often cannot afford the standard prices of even inexpensive restaurants and hotels. The family of one child whom we observed while he was hospitalized for cardiac catheterization at a major university medical center managed by sleeping in their car.

Many families are prevented from participating in the care of their hospitalized children by work and home responsibilities as well as by lack of money. If parent participation in the care of a sick child is considered to be medically beneficial, then the hospital must assume some responsibility for enabling a parent to get to the hospital and for providing facilities once he is there. The main factors preventing parents from spending more time at the hospital are an inability to get babysitters to take care of other siblings at home, inconvenient and expensive transportation to the hospital, and the fear of losing pay or even the job itself if they take time off from work. Although some of the solutions, like providing sick leave for parents if a child is ill, lie outside the jurisdiction of the health care system, much can be done by the individual hospital to help parents get to the hospital when needed by a sick child.

*Design Guidelines*

Provide a hospital jitney service to transport visitors to and from the hospital if public transportation is inconvenient or expensive.

Provide facilities for child care for siblings at or near the hospital. This facility should include a recreation playroom, with a connecting outdoor area if possible, and should be staffed with a child care worker or recreation director. Entrance and exit must be controlled to ensure that children leave only in the company of their parents. Include sleeping areas for a few children, available for 24-hour use, because sick children may be brought to the hospital at any hour of the day.

Provide for an inexpensive parents' hostel within a few minutes walking distance of the hospital. European tourist hostels, boarding houses, and student dormitories provide housing models perhaps more applicable than accommodations currently available.

Provide for inexpensive meal service for families of hospitalized children.

## Provide Internal Facilities for Parent Participation

Most parents will spend some time with their hospitalized children and can be most effective if the hospital is designed with their participation in mind. Internal facilities to accommodate family participation should include places for parents to spend the night, areas in which to prepare food or snacks, to bathe, dress, and play with their child, and space away from the unit for relaxation and rest. Routines should be organized to accommodate parents joining their child at meals and for other common familial activities.

### OVERNIGHT ACCOMMODATIONS

Although it is often advisable for a parent to spend the night with his child, very few hospitals provide space for this purpose. A parent is fortunate if he finds a fold-up cot next to his child's bed. In some hospitals, a parent must sleep in a chair. The lack of adequate facilities for rest exhausts the parent and discourages his participation in the care of his child.

## *Design Guidelines*

Provide a sufficient number of private rooms and baths on each nursing unit to accommodate parents overnight. More such rooms will be needed on units for young children; fewer, if any, in units for adolescents.

Design the space to provide for daybeds, murphy beds, or other comfortable sleeping accommodations.

Provide curtains or other means of obtaining privacy.

Provide storage facilities for parents' clothing.

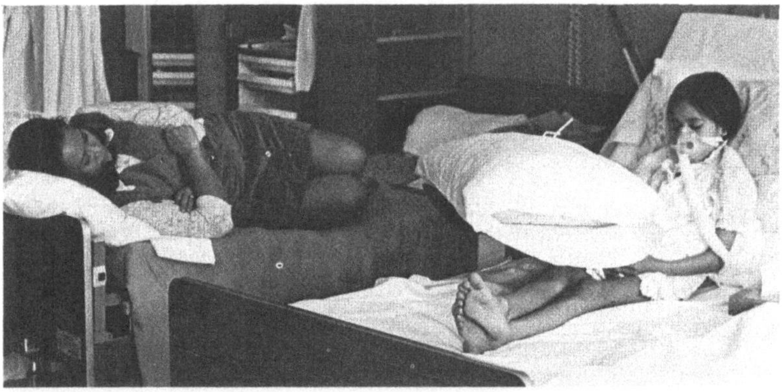

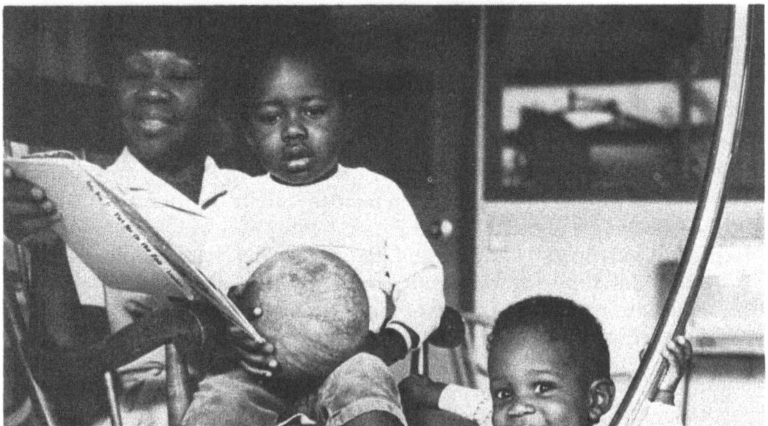

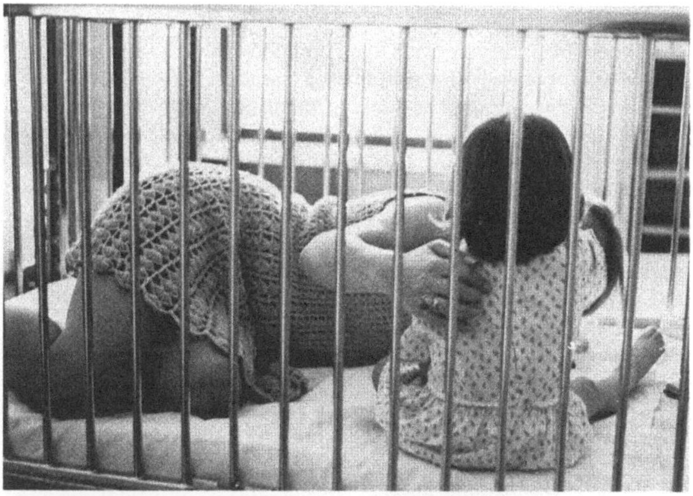

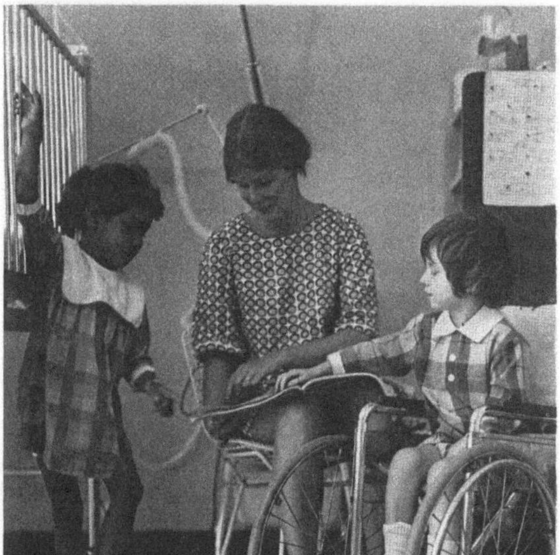

PARENTS' STATION

When parents stay with their child for any length of time, conflicts may arise between the nurses and parents. From the nurses' point of view, the parents may be untidy, incapable of providing hospital nursing care, and annoyingly inactive.[8] The parents thus feel both insecure and unsupported.[9] However, it is unnatural for parents not to participate in the care of their child, particularly a young child. They are used to feeding, changing diapers, making beds, and tidying up. A parent can derive both satisfaction and needed occupation by preparing special meals and snacks for his child. In addition, the preparation of a child's favorite food can encourage him to eat. Children sometimes eat very poorly in the hospital; besides not feeling well, they often have decided food prejudices. Children from diverse cultural groups eat better if served the foods they are used to. Hospital dietary departments are seldom equipped with training or know-how to accommodate diverse food habits. Parents can play an important role in cooking and serving favorite dishes, cookies, and snacks.

In fact, the parents may be considerably more expert about their own child's needs than a nurse. The conflict could be minimized if the hospital would assign a nurses' aide to help parents bathe, dress, and feed their child according to hospital routine, maintain facilities used by parents in neat and clean condition, and act as liaison between parents and professional nurses.[10] Moreover, the hospital should provide a recognized place for parents. The conflict between parents and nurses is exaggerated because of the lack of a territory for parents. Parents need to have their own space both for practical reasons, in order to store equipment and carry out activities without infringing on the nurses' domain or interfering with ongoing operations, and for symbolic reasons, to establish their right to be there.

## *Design Guidelines*

Provide a parents' station on or near the pediatric nursing unit.

Provide sufficient space for two persons to sit down and write. In maintaining accurate records, the parent assumes real responsibility for child care.

Provide storage space for the child's linen, gowns, and diapers.

Provide storage space for records, books, and toys used especially by parents to entertain their children.

Provide food preparation facilities for parents' use.

## Rest and Relaxation Spaces Away from Children

Parents with children in the hospital must have a place to go to relax away from the children. Nurses need time away from children, and such respite is doubly important for parents, who may be under considerable strain. Relaxation for a parent may mean a variety of things: a cigarette, a cup of coffee, a quick nap, a shower to freshen up, a chance for casual conversation with others, a place to escape the surveillance of the staff, or a relaxed place to wait while one's child is undergoing treatment or tests. The provision of toilet and shower facilities for both parents is essential, particularly for the fathers, as mothers can often share the nurses' facilities if no other special provision has been made. Fathers would have greater difficulty in sharing doctors' accommodations.

*Design Guidelines*

Design a lounge to accommodate from five to ten adults. A lounge of this size is comparable to a residential living room and can be a comfortable, informal, noninstitutional place. Larger lounges, such as provided in college dormitories and hotel lobbies, become institutional in character.[11]

Provide facilities for preparation of coffee and simple snacks. Cooking facilities at the parent station could be used for this purpose.

Provide visual distraction. Parents waiting in the lounge for child to return from surgery or from some diagnostic test are often upset. Views outside, wall collages, and paintings can distract a parent and provide needed relaxation.

Provide toilet and shower facilities for both mothers and fathers near but not directly connected to the lounge.

Provide a small area with a comfortable bed for napping near the lounge.

Provide lockable lockers or closet space for parents' coats and a few belongings.

CARE-BY-PARENT UNITS

In most countries of the world, the child does not go to the hospital alone. Rather, the entire family goes to the hospital with the child and cares for his needs.[12] But in the United States, for the parents to live in the hospital and help take care of their children on a full-time basis is a relatively new phenomenon.[13]

In care-by-parent units, one or both parents enter the hospital with their sick child, perhaps with his healthy siblings as well, prepared to perform many nursing functions.[14] The type of care rendered by parents varies in different settings. In some units, in addition to bathing, feeding, and entertaining a child, parents take urine samples and temperatures or give medications and injections.[15]

In addition to reducing the trauma of separation and hospitalization, advocates of care-by-parent units claim other important advantages. For example, the child may be able to go home sooner if the parent has had instruction in caring for him. The cost of pediatric care may be lowered if the parent carries out tasks that would normally require staff time.[16] Physicians, nurses, and students can benefit from the opportunity to observe and evaluate parent-child interaction. Finally, contact with other parents of sick children can provide parents with needed support.[17]

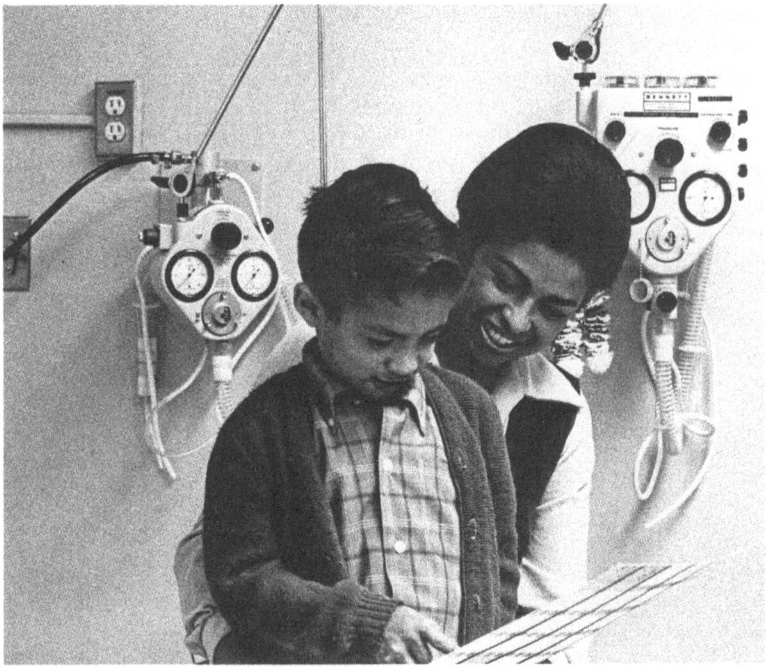

*Family Participation*

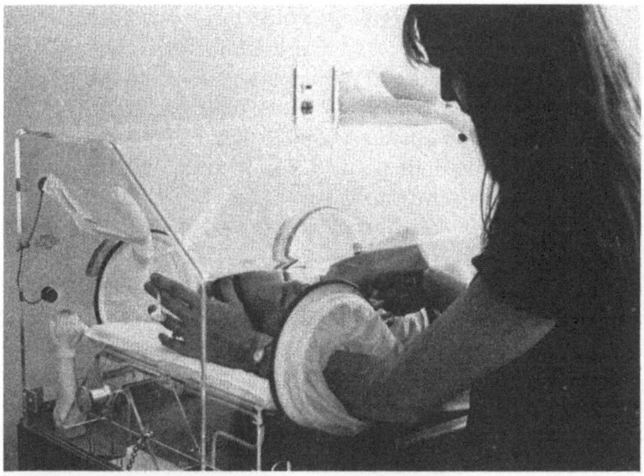

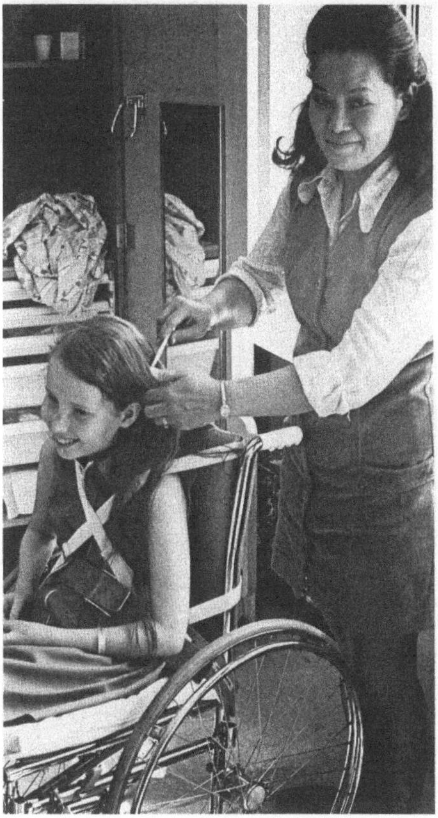

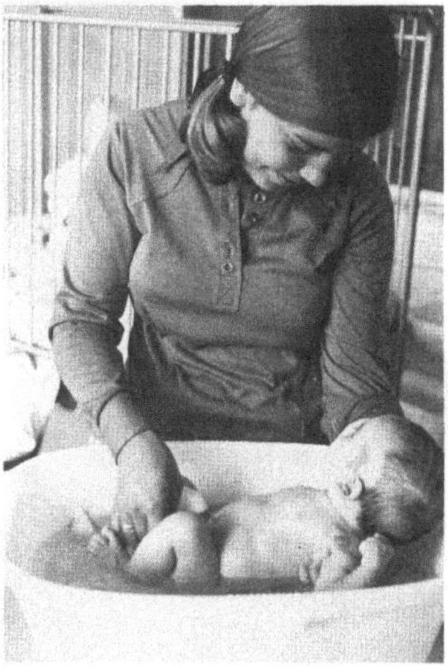

The ability for parents to support each other, however, is dependent on their ability to communicate with each other. Some nurses, doctors, and parents themselves believe that parental participation creates more work for nurses rather than less, that parents often upset their children, and that better nursing care is given by trained personnel than by parents.[18] These negative attitudes are generated in part by the newness of the concept and by the difference in approach from the traditional hospital pattern, in which authority for a child is transferred on admission from the parent to the nurse.[19]

In British live-in programs, moreover, where mothers are relieved of all household responsibilities, it is reported that they become desperately bored. They are placed in the unnatural situation of being in constant and close contact with their child for twenty-four hours a day. Normally both mother and child have many independent activities. A mother keeps house, shops, walks, and visits with friends. In turn, a child plays with other children, visits relatives, goes to nursery school, and functions for periods of time without his mother. In the hospital situation the normal mother-child situation is altered. The result of a lack of work and the unnatural amount of time devoted solely to her child may cause a woman to "look forward to discharge from the hospital as if to the end of a long prison sentence."[20] Part of the success of parent participation programs will therefore depend on the facilities provided for the individual parent and child, as well as on the facilities and arrangements for group interaction. Despite all the difficulties, the option to stay with and care for his child should be provided a parent.

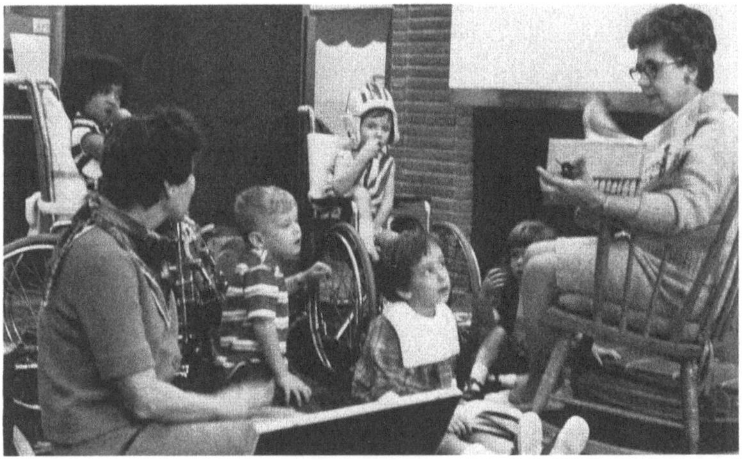

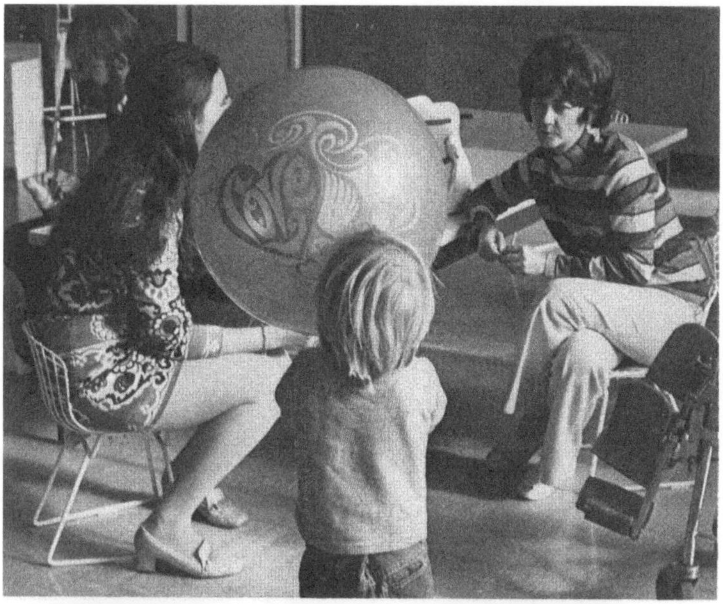

*Family Participation*

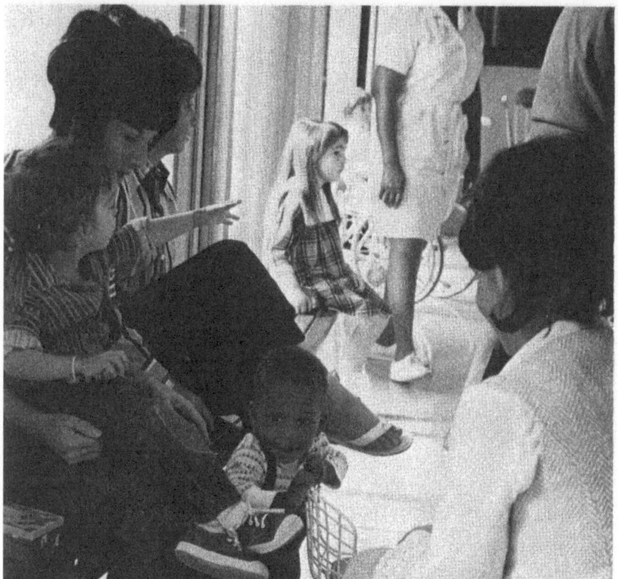

## *Design Guidelines*

Provide stipends for parents who wish to assume nursing responsibility but are financially unable to. Some hospitals find that savings in nursing costs justify this expense.

Model the care-by-parent unit after a home for a very large family, with a separate room and bath for each patient and parent, and group space for socializing, preparation of snacks, laundry, and storage.

Limit the capacity of the unit to no more than eight patients so that the families can comfortably share a large family-like lounge, kitchen facilities, and laundry. If too many people use these facilities, the regulations required to coordinate their use and to keep them clean tend to negate the informal atmosphere desired. Even assuming that several families will spend much time confined to their rooms, more than eight child-parent residents is too large a group for them to get to know and help each other easily.

Locate the care-by-parent unit near the acute pediatric unit, so as to have immediate access to professional nurses and staff physicians and special equipment. Children will often be transferred from more intensive professional care in the pediatric unit to the care-by-patient unit or the reverse.

Design the facility so that a parent can watch a child at play and still prepare a snack, do chores, or rest, as he would at home.

Design the room for patient and family to function as a living room as well as a bedroom. Provide sufficient space to accommodate both parents and siblings, if necessary.

# The Staff 8

The needs of the pediatric patient can be met only if the requirements for equipment, space, work flow, interaction, relaxation, and job satisfaction of the medical and paramedical staff are also met effectively. At the turn of the century the nurse took care of almost all patient needs. Today patient-care functions have been subdivided into service functions, medical functions, and administrative functions. Each of these in turn is provided by a variety of different types of personnel. Children in hospitals regularly come into contact with both practical and registered nurses, aides and orderlies, staff physicians and medical house officers. A lab technician takes a child's blood; an x-ray technician photographs his body; a physical therapist manipulates his limbs. Psychiatrists, psychologists, and social workers assess his emotional well-being. Occupational therapists, recreational directors, child care workers, school teachers, visitors, and volunteers meet his nonmedical needs. Janitors, service men, housekeepers, and maids keep his room clean and the equipment in repair. His food is planned by the dietitian, delivered by food servers, and eaten sometimes with other children. In fact, one four-year-old child who was observed in a modern, highly respected medical institution came into visual and social contact with twenty-five different persons within a three-hour period.

Each of these occupational groups has a function to perform and requires both equipment and space. In addition, each of these persons needs a place for relaxation and for interaction with others. People unhappy in their job environment will take it out directly or indirectly on the children. All requirements must be evaluated within the context of the child's needs.

A primary need of the child is to feel at home with an understanding and empathetic staff. This condition often depends on shared ethnic and cultural patterns, which can affect everything from dietary habits to norms for child raising and names for body parts. Bilingualism is crucial in many communities. Some children communicate best with nonprofessional staff or volunteers from their own community. Unfortunately, these nonprofessionals are seldom fully included in decision-making and coordinating health care.

## Encourage Communication and Teamwork

Staff interaction and communication must be fostered. Although the physical facility cannot bridge the social gulfs created and maintained by the rigid organizational structure of the hospital, it can provide opportunities for easy formal and informal interaction.

With so many persons involved in the care of the child, it would seem obvious that various staff members should coordinate their work. Yet "one of the biggest and most universal hospital problems [is] getting the staff to work together." [1] A major reason for this difficulty can be traced to the vast differences in social status among different staff members.

The hospital has its roots in the hierarchical and authoritarian organization of religious orders and military institutions, and much of the same structure still prevails. Today, the doctor is probably the most authoritarian figure, although to some extent he shares this position with administrators and boards of trustees. Within the nursing system, the registered nurse has the greatest prestige, then the vocational nurse, finally the nurses' aide. At the lowest level of the social pyramid are the service personnel — janitors, cleaning women, and food servers.[2] This stratification is reinforced by a system that rarely allows promotion from one level to another (L.V.N. to R.N., R.N. to M.D.) and by ethnic and linguistic differences among the levels that tend to restrict communication. Efforts have been made to alter the structure so that true team function will result, but the most difficult concept for all organizations to recognize is that "the best team is not just a collection of the people who have the most skill as individuals, but of people with high individual skill who can also work well together." [3]

### PARTICIPATION BY ALL SUBGROUPS WITHIN COMMUNITY

The stratification that inhibits effective teamwork also plays a part in inhibiting full community involvement in the dispensing of health care. Pediatric units have long been the province of white, middle-class women. Because children communicate more fully with staff members from similar backgrounds, it is essential that minority staff members and male staff members be recruited through volunteer and paid summer internship programs for adolescents, foster grandparent programs, job training and new career programs, alternative service programs for conscientious objectors to the draft, and any other means available to interest a broad cross-section of the community in health work.

*Design Guidelines*

Provide teaching and volunteer agency space in the hospital for programs to recruit and train community workers. Neighborhood health centers could provide initial recruitment and education and familiarize interested persons with the job possibilities in health.

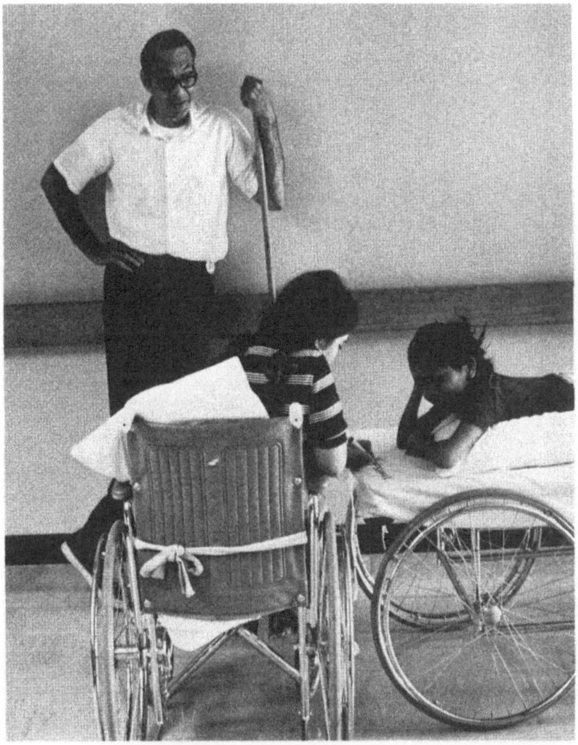

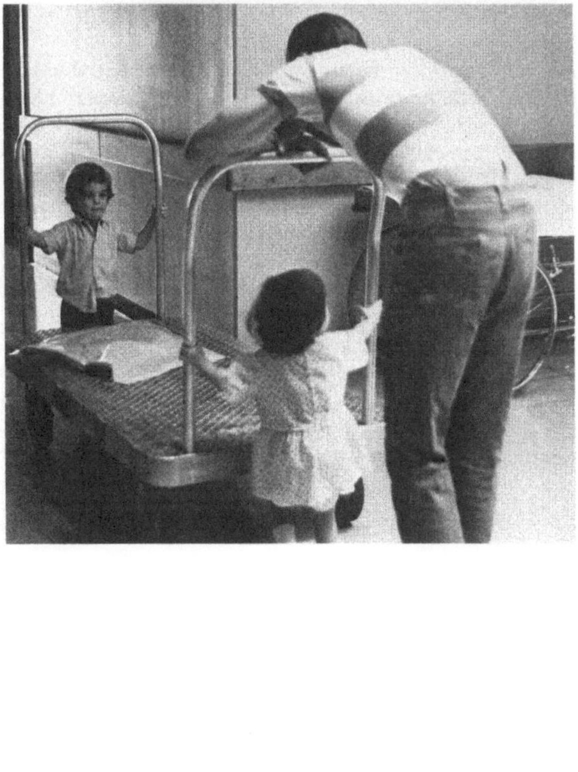

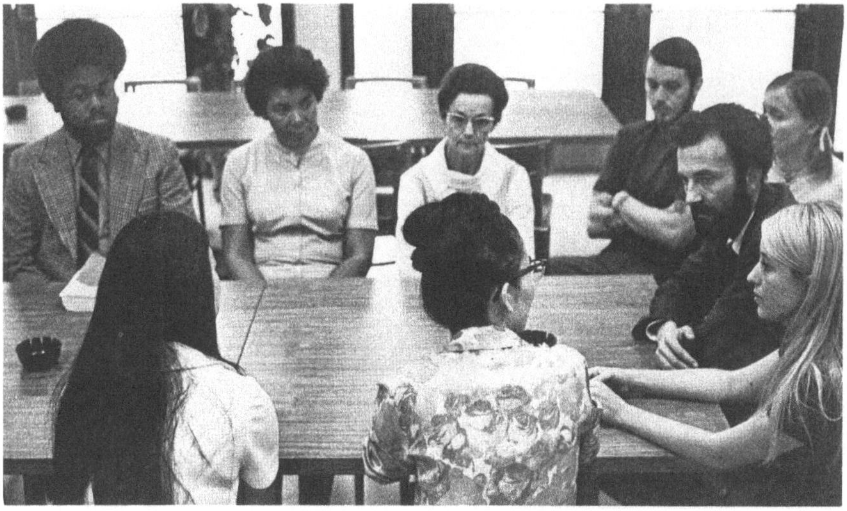

## TEAM MEETING ROOMS

One way for a staff to begin to develop a sense of "team" is to hold regular meetings of all persons involved in the care of specific children. Efforts are being made in many pediatric institutions to hold unit "team meetings" to discuss problems of patient care, discipline, and behavior. The setting for such meetings should provide an atmosphere conducive to the exchange of ideas between all personnel, regardless of status position.

### *Design Guidelines*

Provide a meeting place near the pediatric unit to accommodate from six to twelve persons. Research into the group size most effective for maximum participation suggests that the ideal discussion group consists of about twelve persons. If the group gets larger, general experience in university seminars, club meetings, and other conference situations has shown that fewer individuals participate. The session tends to become a lecture or is monopolized by a few people. Decision-making is slowed, which forces ranking members to exert influence.

Locate the meeting place near the pediatric unit so that those working there can attend more easily and still be within call. A conveniently located, attractive room can function as a locus for informal contact among team workers as well.

Furnish the room with a round table and comfortable chairs. Since round tables have no head, there is less possibility for individuals to reinforce status positions through seating location. A round table also allows all the people to see one another.[4]

Provide a coffee pot to produce a more relaxed and pleasant atmosphere.

Soundproof the room so that children cannot hear what is going on.

Equip the room with blackboards, tack boards, and x-ray boxes for demonstration and display.

## Increase Patient Contact and Job Satisfaction for Nurses

Present-day nursing practice grew out of the need for someone to take care of the feeding, bathing, toileting, and other requirements of patients in the hospital. Many women went into nursing because of the satisfactions gained from caring for patients who were helpless and in need. As medical treatment advanced in complexity, the nurse took on many tasks requiring a high degree of technical and medical skill. The nursing function, in addition to providing for the physical and emotional needs of the patient, required education in medical techniques and procedures. Today there are three types of hospital employees generally called nurse — the registered nurse or R.N., who generally has completed three years of nursing school, the licensed practical nurse (called licensed vocational nurse or L.V.N. in some states), who has a year of training, and the nurses' aide or orderly, who generally has no formal training other than that received on the job.

In the 1950's and 1960's, changes developed in the roles ascribed to nursing personnel, as scores of functions formerly performed by registered nurses or nursing students were "allocated to practical nurses, aides, ward secretaries, maids, cleaning men, persons who transport food trays."[5] The theory was that the more the nurse was freed from "menial" tasks, the more she would have time for the sophisticated nursing services.

Architects cooperated in this effort in a number of ways. First, they tried to design nursing units that would reduce the number of steps a nurse had to walk, again on the theory that the time saved in walking would be devoted to patient care. The nursing unit with the least distance from the nursing station to the most remote bedroom door was considered to be the most efficient and thus became the primary design goal. Further studies on nursing efficiency revealed that a nurse's travel pattern could more truly be measured by the cumulative distance of all the trips she made. For a period of time, the Yale index, a method devised for this type of efficiency evaluation, was the hospital architect's bible.[6] The second most influential criterion affecting nursing unit planning was the concept that increased size and more centralized service equaled greater efficiency.

Paradoxically, the efforts made to increase nurses' job efficiency resulted in a lowering of the quality of patient care. "The present system of subdivision of labor that begins to resemble the assembly line of an industrial plant, appears to yield satisfaction neither for many of the staff nor for a considerable proportion of the patients. It has also failed to yield the degree of hoped-for efficiency." [7]

Today there is talk of a nurse shortage crisis. However, research into the facts behind the nurse shortage reveals that in terms of absolute figures, "the number of professional nurses per 100 beds in 1964 was almost four times as great as in 1941, and 50 percent more than in 1952." [8] The problem is obviously not really a shortage of nurses, but rather the fact that many registered nurses are not practicing. Among those who do practice there is a high turnover and low productivity.

The rapid turnover at all levels of hospital nursing staff indicates a basic dissatisfaction among registered nurses, licensed practical nurses, nurse's aides, and orderlies.[9] The reasons given for this turnover include low wages, awkward working hours, limited opportunities for advancement, difficult working relations created by the hospital bureaucratic and authoritarian system, lack of a clearly-defined job function, and sex discrimination.[10]

Many nurses choose nursing as a profession because they want to care for the sick. Under current circumstances, the registered nurse spends most of her time coordinating the activity of the diverse personnel involved in different aspects of patient care or in giving medication and specific treatments, which leaves her inadequate time to spend with a child.[11] As for the nurses' aide and licensed vocational nurse, work on the nursing unit has been so subdivided that the jobs hold little interest. There is little or no prestige attached to the work nor is there room for advancement.[12] As one observer reported, "if nursing aides have often concluded that they were 'low men on the totem pole' the behavior of their immediate bosses and also of the staff nurses has frequently justified that conclusion," whereas registered nurses "resented the fact that even some of their duties could be performed by women and men who had very brief training." [13]

The low-status position of licensed vocational nurses, aides and orderlies is reinforced by a lack of physical territory. The head nurse has a private office; the registered nurses work out of nurses' stations. The transients on the nursing unit, such as radiology and laboratory technicians, physical and occupational therapists, all have a home territory in their own departments. Territory identifies a person with a place, and creates a sense of belonging, yet no place is provided for the majority of the nursing staff.[14]

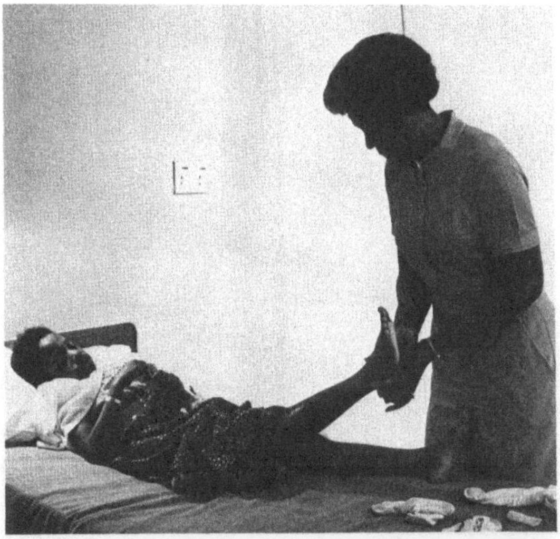

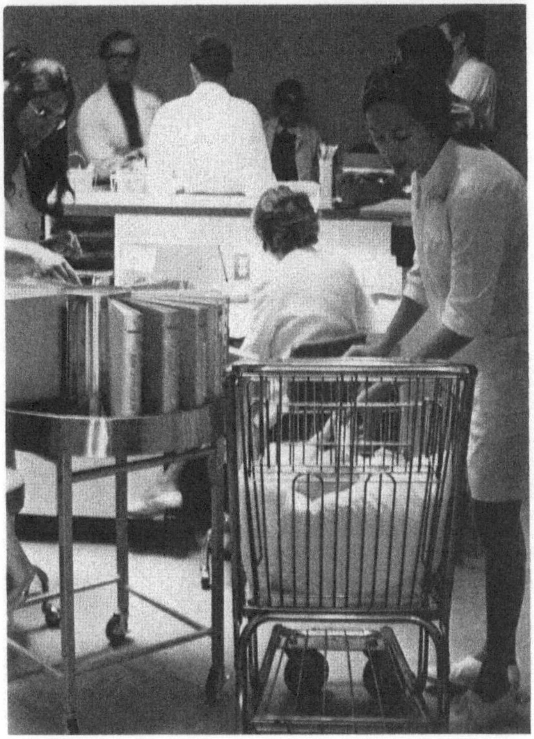

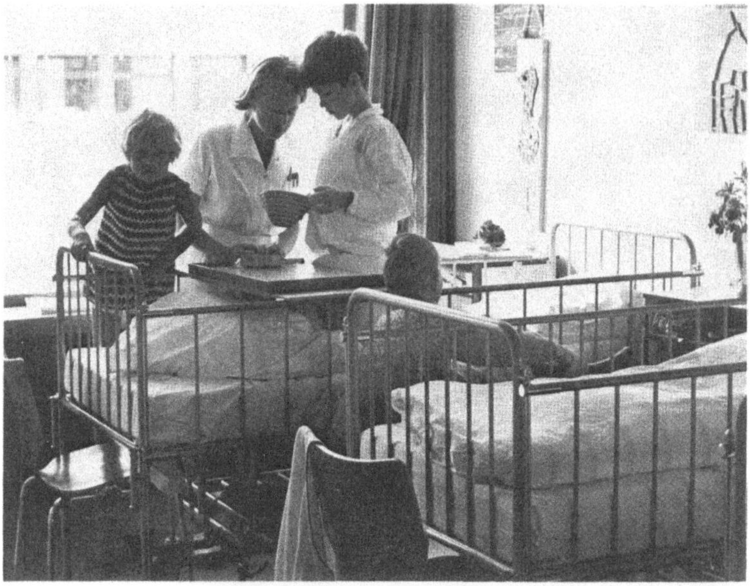

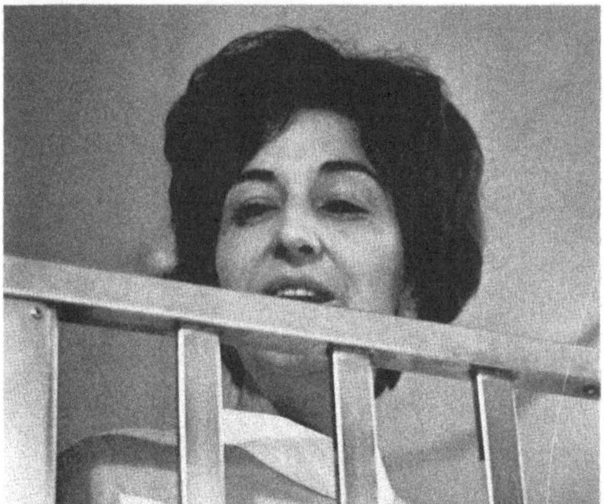

Most people require and thrive on informal relations within their occupational group. A pediatric nurse, in particular, cannot spend her entire work day with her young patients. She needs adult, professional contact to keep up with the latest nursing techniques, to discuss the children's problems, to relax from the tensions of dealing with very ill or dying children and their families, and to develop needed social relations. The nursing staff has difficulty in developing these needed group relations, owing to the problems of part-time assignments, irregular shifts, and high turnover.[15]

It should be possible to restructure many of the functions performed by licensed vocational nurses, nurses' aides, maids, housekeepers, and food servers into one category called "bedside nurse." If the work and facilities were properly organized, it would be possible for such a person to stay with a small group of children almost continuously, assisted by a nurses' aide. Instead of the relatively low status role currently played by the practical nurse, the bedside nurse could have a unique and valued place on a health team with more highly trained professionals. In addition, this job could provide much greater satisfaction than any of the functions taken separately, and might slow the very high turnover among the semiskilled workers.

The status of the registered nurse must also be raised. Today, many nurses administer complicated medical treatment and in effect often act for the physician. Yet this work is not recognized and adequately rewarded. Esther Brown has described the system of "multiple subordination" which gives the registered nurse considerable responsibility while placing her in a position subordinate to a large variety of other staff members, including other nurses. In short, the registered nurse is too highly trained to allow her to spend her time "nursing," while the licensed vocational nurses and nurses' aides are not considered trained enough to allow them to assume full responsibility for a child. Dissatisfactions related to low status situations and territorial identification compound this problem.

## *Design Guidelines*

Reorganize the nursing station into substations staffed by a "bedside nurse" and aide, responsible for from four to eight patients.

Provide work and storage space at each substation. The notion of a decentralized supply unit was developed and used by Gordon Friesen, who utilized a nurseserver at each room, which contained space for clean and dirty linen and individual medical supplies such as intravenous solutions, hypodermic needles, and syringes.

Organize the substations so that bedside nurses can be in

direct visual contact with children at all times. In the case of older children and adolescents, this option might be used only for patients requiring close observation.

Provide a medical nursing station staffed by a registered nurse, serving several substations but also directly related to a group of children so that this unit is not isolated from direct patient care.

Design the one medical station to contain specialized medical facilities for several subunits. These facilities include space for medication preparation, for storage of drugs and other supplies, and for informal consultation. Depending on the overall nursing unit organization, the medical station might also include the examination-treatment and utility rooms.

Organize the records and communication system so that the medical station can be used to service several substations on off-hours. James Souder and Philip Bonnet developed a clustered plan for adults in the Union Memorial Hospital in Baltimore, in which the nursing unit size differs according to whether it is the day or night shift.

Provide lounge and locker space for pediatric staff outside the pediatric unit.

## Conserve Time of Physicians

The organization and participation of the medical staff within the hospital varies widely: "Some physicians may be attached to the staff of one hospital; others to four or five. Some may spend only a small part of their professional lives in the hospital; others almost all." Some hospitals, particularly teaching hospitals and medical centers, are increasingly developing full-time medical staffs. Community hospitals rely primarily or solely on an attending staff whose members spend several hours a day in the hospital. However, in teaching hospitals, "with ever-growing patient loads, attending doctors are relying more and more heavily on interns and residents to help care for their hospitalized patients . . . Although the number of interns and residents has grown strikingly in recent years, it has fallen far short of the demand. Moreover, American-trained interns and residents will not now go to hospitals . . . where there is little or no educational opportunity. The situation in some hospitals has reached crisis proportions." [16]

Typically, a doctor spends his time on a nursing unit in visiting his patient, checking the charts, consulting with the nursing staff, examining and treating the patient, issuing orders for medication, dictating, talking to patients and their families, and teaching. The doctor's time is a scarce and expensive commodity. The anxiety of treating very ill children and particularly the necessity of making life-and-death decisions under extreme time pressure indicate the need to place a high premium on environmental features that might save minutes, relax the pace of a doctor's day, and allow him to relate more meaningfully to staff, patients, and parents.

Doctors are often held in awe, so that nonphysicians sometimes hesitate to try to talk with them. Yet in some instances a few words with a doctor would alleviate fears and tension, particularly in adolescents wanting an opportunity to find out what is wrong with them, who would come to a consultation room if it were readily accessible.

The private physician or specialist often has his patients scattered throughout the hospital, with the result that much of his time is spent between patients rather than with them. This is one reason that some physicians prefer grouping patients by disease categories rather than by age groups. Examination, treatment, teaching, and consultation are carried out at the patient's bedside, generally because of lack of time. Even though an examination-treatment room is usually provided on each nursing unit, the experience of most hospitals indicates that they are seldom used for the purpose intended. They become instead additional storage areas.

There are many opinions as to the most desirable location for a treatment room. Some say it should be located on each nursing unit and be visible to the other children, as the worst that they will witness is infinitely less terrifying than the horrors they imagine. Others advocate that the examination-treatment room be away from the unit and be soundproofed, so that no one hears or sees what is going on.

It takes less time for a doctor to examine a patient in bed than in an examining room, and in many cases it may be better for the patient not to be moved. However, if the bed is used for painful examinations and procedures, it loses its value as a place of safety and refuge and may cause emotional problems for the child. A refusal to relax or sleep in bed may be traceable to this practice.

Doctors frequently conduct consultations in the corridor, where parents and children may overhear parts of the conversation. Some doctors recognize the harmful effects of this practice, but their busy schedules seldom permit the use of a consultation room away from the immediate vicinity.

There has been an increasing trend for doctors to locate their offices in or near hospitals because of the advantages offered by close proximity to diagnostic and therapeutic services and travel time saved.[17] From the physician's point of view the ideal physical configuration would provide

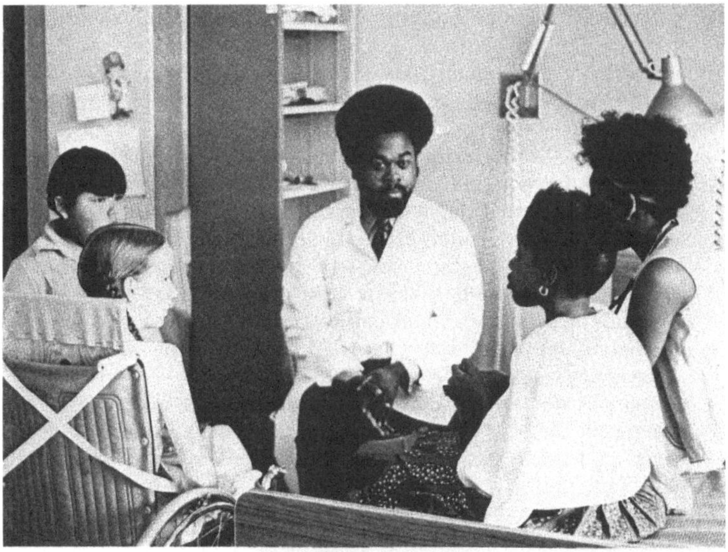

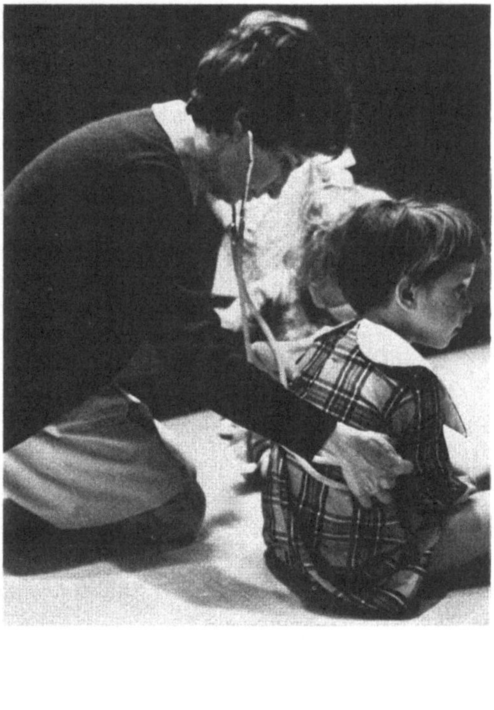

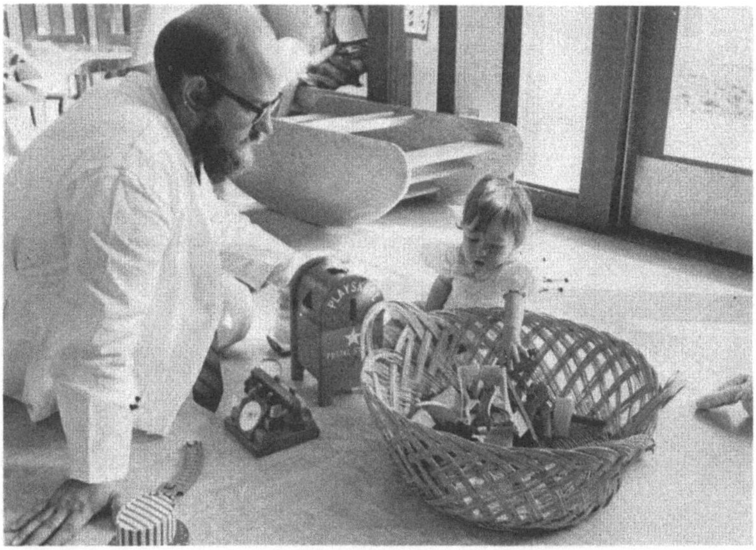

contiguous facilities for his bed patients, his ambulant patients, his teaching activities, and his research endeavors. For the house officer, the closer his quarters are to the pediatric unit, the more likely he will be to spend time becoming comfortably familiar with its patients, staff, and operations, and the better prepared he will be to make decisions appropriate to each highly individualized situation.

## *Design Guidelines*

Provide facilities close-by for a resident staff of house officers. This should include offices, personal storage space, lounge areas, and overnight accommodations for both male and female residents and interns.

Provide an examination-treatment, consultation, and demonstration room complex serving several nursing units. The number of examination-treatment and consultation rooms will vary with the type of pediatric patient, the number of patients per horizontal level, the degree of illness, and the type of treatment rendered. In some instances, it would be possible to use these rooms for outpatients as well as for inpatients.

Provide two examination-treatment rooms for every consultation room so that a physician will not be kept waiting for a patient.

Make the examination-treatment rooms sufficiently large to accommodate a patient bed or gurney in addition to the examination table.

Soundproof the examination-treatment and consultation rooms.

Design the consultation rooms to be informal and conducive to sharing confidences. There is less formality if the patient or patient's family sits alongside the doctor rather than faces him over a desk.

Provide visual aides in the consultation room to explain particular disease problems.

Provide dictating equipment, x-ray view boxes, and convenient writing space to make the most of the doctor's time while he is present.

Make the consultation room easily accessible from the corridor without going through other space.

## Provide Opportunities for Students on the Nursing Unit

Many hospitals today serve as the locus of a teaching function as well as for rendering medical care. Students in training include doctors, medical students, nurses, technicians, therapists, and other groups of medical, paramedical, and service personnel. The presence of students representing so many different disciplines, particularly within the teaching hospital, generates a need for more space than would typically be required for most patient care functions per se.

Students participate in large lectures, small seminar meetings, medical rounds, informal sessions, and one-to-one patient contact. In addition, they require space to store their belongings, to study and meet. Although space for most of these functions is provided off the nursing unit, the students, particularly nursing and medical students, come to the nursing unit daily to participate in medical rounds.

Historically, clinical training has been provided by the professor making rounds with his students. This pattern still remains, with groups of nurses and medical students following one or more instructors from bed to bed. In the design of teaching hospitals, architects are schooled to provide space around the patient's bed, the examination room, and the surgical theater large enough to accommodate the teacher and student population.

The system of hospital rounding is well entrenched in daily patient care routine. Yet from the child's view, "these rounds are one of the most

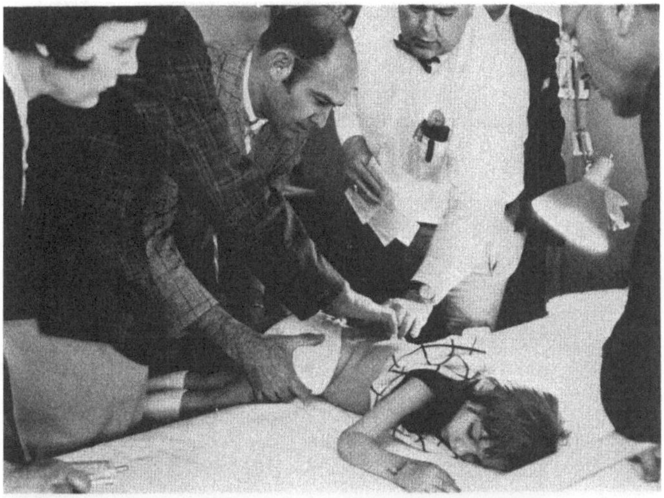

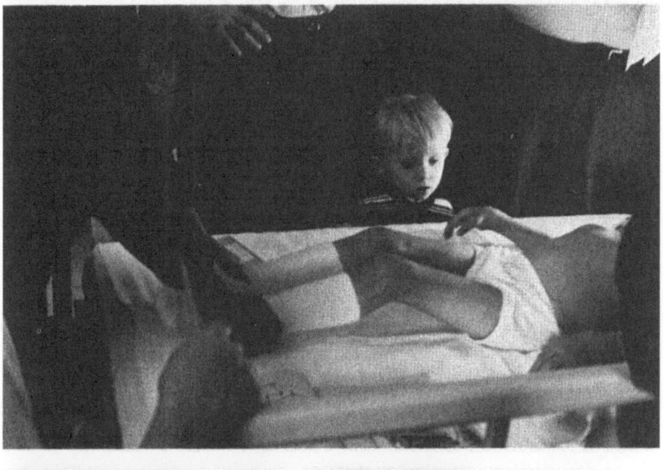

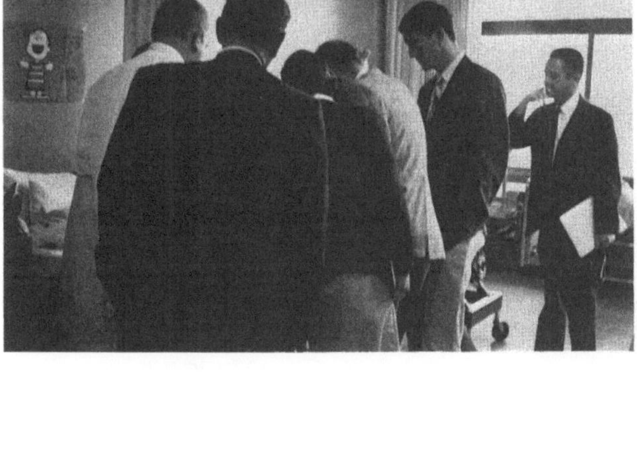

threatening and traumatic experiences he suffers during hospitalization. The child looks at the group and recognizes only one or two faces. The people are dressed in white, are quite serious, and talk in terms he cannot understand. Sometimes the outlook and prognosis of the child is discussed at this time . . . From the point of view of the emotional and social well-being of the children, these rounds should be abandoned." [18] At the very minimum, teaching rounds present a child with exposure to a confusingly large number of strange adults, less expert and often painful handling, and embarrassing exposure and infringement of privacy, particularly if the examination occurs in multibed rooms. For example, an adolescent with a bladder disease was observed being examined in turn by five medical students and their clinical instructor. Each then offered his diagnosis. Those suggesting appendicitis and lower back ailments were asked to examine her abdomen again. The entire process was conducted behind a curtain, with two adolescent roommates listening the whole time.

## *Design Guidelines*

Provide a closed-circuit TV system at each patient's bed and in the examination-treatment demonstration room, which eliminates the necessity for large groups converging on a youngster.

Connect the TV system to viewing rooms throughout the hospital.

Record every examination and treatment procedure on video tape, so as to provide a visual record of the progress of the patient.

Make the demonstration room large enough to accommodate a patient in his bed.

Provide raised observation space along an entire wall, with one-way mirrors looking into the demonstration room.

Provide small meeting rooms near each pediatric unit for informal discussion between students and faculty.

Provide additional space as needed to allow students to observe or participate in specified functions, such as charting and medicine preparation, without interfering with the efficiency of the work environment.

# The Pediatric Nursing Unit 9

The design of the nursing unit determines the design of the hospital. Decisions regarding the size and organization of nursing units, the ways in which patients and their families are grouped, the facilities and criteria required by these groupings, and the relationships of the nursing units to each other critically influence the design of the entire hospital complex and reflect program definition as well as personnel and patient needs.

Since World War II the nursing unit design has been influenced by the concept that size and centralization are essential to efficient operation. For a decade nursing units have progressively increased in size from about twenty beds to over sixty. The past five years have seen a general reaction against both size and centralization. The theoretical efficiency attributed to centralization and increased size is being questioned and has assumed less value when measured on a scale that places a higher premium on the patient's sense of security and well-being. Today there is a marked trend toward planning the nursing unit so as to bring the nurse into closer contact with the patient, and it is anticipated that there will be greater efforts to adjust the hospital environment to the needs of individual children of all ages and developmental levels.

## Size

Many factors of size determine the design of a nursing unit: the size most conducive to peer group interaction, most efficient for nursing team care, permitting maximum direct visual supervision, encouraging close nurse-patient relationships, and making most economical use of specialized equipment and services. The Platt Report states that "it should be possible to run children's wards with as few as eight to ten beds," and that, "this number would justify the appointment of a sick children's trained nurse." [1] The American Academy of Pediatrics recommends "no fewer than 14 beds and no more than 24." [2] The Children's Hospital at Stanford provides fourteen beds per unit, while the Kaiser Foundation Hospital in Walnut Creek, California, has eight beds to a nursing station. The Boston Floating

Hospital study recommends ten-bed units, a smaller number for intensive care, and a larger number for adolescents.[3] Emma Plank reports that ten beds in a long-term tuberculosis unit works well for grade school children.[4] The Nuffield Foundation in England recommends a unit of twenty beds based on availability of trained staff and staffing patterns in England.[5]

*Design Guidelines*

Plan nursing subunits to accommodate four beds for infants, six to eight beds for toddlers and preschoolers, twelve beds for grade school children, and eight to twenty-four beds for adolescents.

## Grouping

Patients can be grouped according to age, disease, treatment needs, income, ethnic group, sex, intensity of illness, or length of stay. Historically, children were cared for on the women's medical wards, where they were exposed to unpleasant sights and situations that they could not handle. Today, no one recommends mixing children and adults in any but the most exceptional circumstances, such as in the case of an accident or epidemic causing several members of the same family to be hospitalized simultaneously.

Grouping by disease pattern is still sometimes recommended because the opportunities to treat large numbers of patients with similar disease patterns have led to a greater understanding of the physiological and psychological effects of certain diseases and greater skill in treating patients. In addition, specialized staff and equipment can be provided, and children gain support from knowing others with similar medical problems. Recommendations for continued grouping by intensity of illness are based on the savings in cost achieved by concentrating needed, skilled personnel and equipment, and on the better nursing care achieved by locating intensely ill patients in close proximity to specialized equipment and personnel. Separation by length of stay is advocated on the grounds that long-term patients find the admission, recovery, and departure for home of short-term patients discouraging and depressing; special facilities can be provided for long-term care in the form of schools and recreational facilities; and specialized staff are needed for long-term rehabilitative care.

Today, however, though some still suggest grouping pediatric patients on the basis of disease, intensity of illness, or length of stay, most pediatricians, child psychiatrists, and psychologists believe grouping by age to be the most beneficial arrangement for the social and emotional well-being of the child. The most effective care, programs, facilities, and peer group relationships can be accomplished if children are grouped according to age level.[6]

Age grouping should not be followed inflexibly, however. Any pediatric department, whether the specific grouping pattern is by age, disease, or intensity of illness, will find it extremely difficult to predict and plan admissions so as to maintain grouping categories. Inevitably, there will be a greater demand for beds in one group than in another. Without sufficient flexibility to provide for variation in the size of each nursing unit or subunit to accommodate these shifts in demand, the hospital will be forced either to refuse admissions or to accommodate patients in environments unsuited to their age needs. A teenager could find himself adjacent to a sick elderly man; a ten-year-old could be heartbroken to find himself with a group of toddlers.

Perhaps the requirement most often stated by doctors and administrators is that the building be flexible. Flexibility has many interpretations, which range from the ability to create a "university space" adaptable for any purpose to more limited concepts that include the ability to move a wall or relocate a door. Very flexible buildings, such as offices and laboratories, have been developed to provide large unbroken spaces with movable partitions and continuous access to water, electricity, air conditioning, and other services. In laboratories and hospitals such flexibility has been achieved by providing alternate floors designed solely to accommodate ducts, pipes, conduit, and equipment. Although this type of flexibility is expensive, it is appropriate for facilities requiring constant changes in equipment. It is unwarranted for nursing units, which have undergone little basic change over the years. The degree of flexibility needed in most buildings can be more simply provided by using a hung ceiling and allowing access to the resulting service space.

The type of flexibility desired also varies with the time and scope of change required. Instant flexibility is sometimes needed, as in transforming a gymnasium into a cafeteria at lunch time. Long-term flexibility is desirable if the need arises, for example, to knock out and relocate walls without destroying the structural integrity of the building. Still another form of flexibility is achieved by careful architectural planning to provide the opportunity to expand a function into adjacent spaces without requiring major structural alterations. This type of flexibility is often most relevant, as building users seldom totally redesign their facility or require expensive instant flexibility, but often need to interchange spaces.

## *Design Guidelines*

Provide special nursing units or subunits for infants, for toddlers, for preschoolers, for school age children, and for teenagers.

Design each nursing unit to overlap with the next unit so that approximately one-third of its beds may be affiliated with either unit. Thus, if the nursing unit optimally contains eight to ten patients, it might potentially include as many as twelve or fourteen beds or as few as six. Overlapping each unit with several other units will maximize flexibility.

Provide loosely defined boundaries between age groups to allow for easy communication and interaction as well as to create opportunities for older children to care for younger ones.

Design bedrooms that can be converted from single to double, and from double to four-bed rooms.

Design the multipurpose space in each nursing unit in the form of a central area surrounded by at least two alcoves easily adaptable for use by all age groups.

Eliminate built-in furniture so that, depending on demand, the furniture most suitable for each age group can be brought in as needed.

Put windows in all interior walls. Visibility can be assured in the case of young children, and privacy can be obtained by the use of curtains for adults or older children.

Design windows and doors that both a young child and an adult can use.

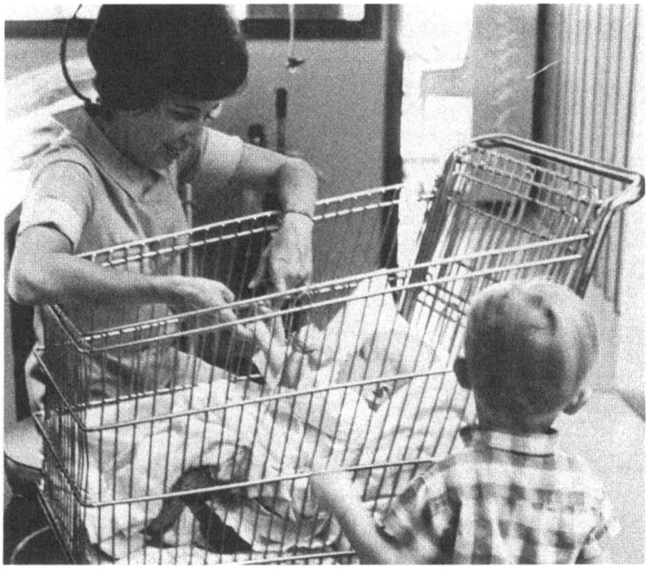

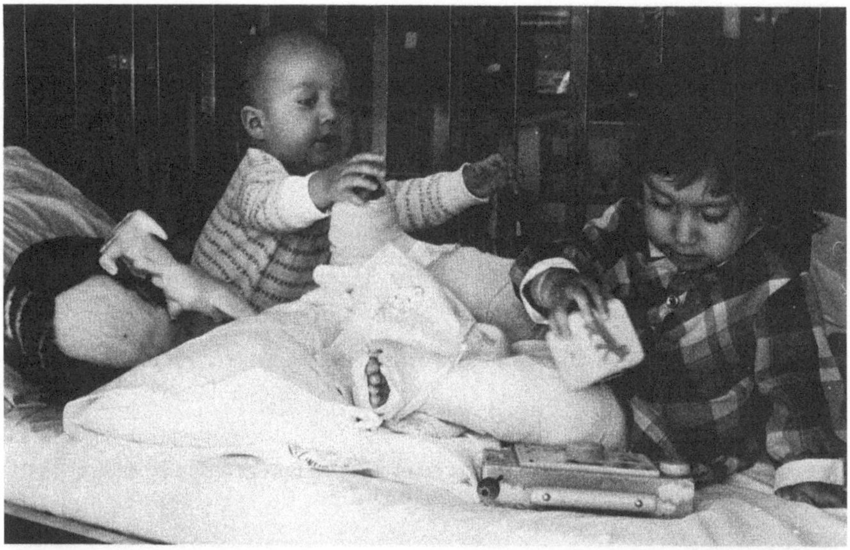

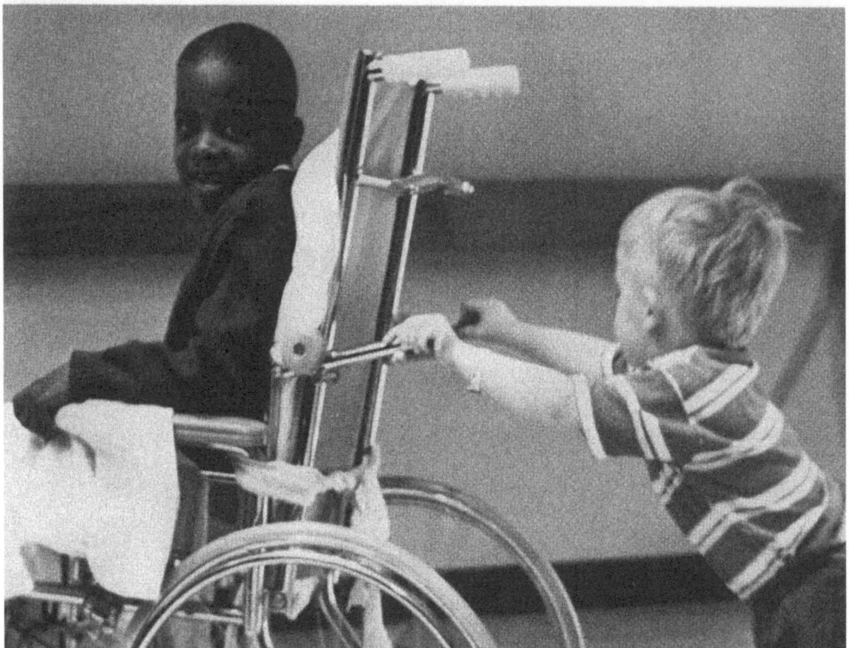

## Shared Use of Specialized Facilities

Certain facilities, if conveniently located, can be used jointly by several nursing units. These include parent facilities, doctors' offices and quarters, examination space, teaching facilities, and conference rooms. Convenience is generally equated with being on the same horizontal level, but successful relationships can be developed between levels if access is easy and clear.

### *Design Guidelines*

Cluster two to four nursing units so as to share in the use of the less heavily used facilities provided for parents, physicians, and medical students.

Arrange parent facilities, doctors' quarters, and lounges so that persons need not pass through a nursing unit to get to them.

Arrange control points for maximum visibility over the entrance to each unit.

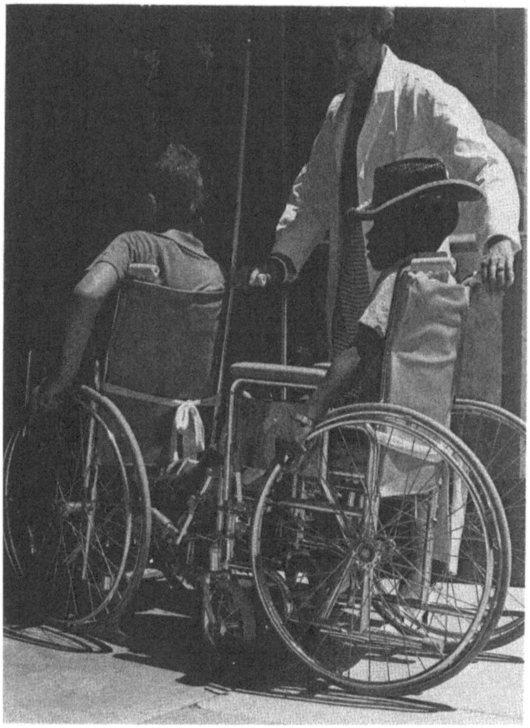

## Access to the Outdoors

With the lessening of febrile, infectious diseases, the need to keep hospitalized children indoors is no longer a general rule. A close relationship between the nursing unit and outdoor areas allows outdoor play to take its natural place in the daily activities of hospital life.

### *Design Guidelines*

Locate pediatric nursing units adjacent to ground floor space that can be developed as a play area.

In crowded urban areas, where play space on the ground is not available, locate the pediatric nursing units adjacent to roof areas that can be developed as play areas.

## Nursing Unit Topology

The functional requirements of the different age groups, of families, and of staff have so far been defined, and design guidelines presented based on these requirements, including general provisions for a distinct territory for each age level, accommodation for parents, separate personal space as well as community space for patients, parents, and staff, a close relationship to the out-of-doors, direct visual supervision, and opportunities for growth and contraction of size. It is now possible to examine the topology of the nursing unit in terms of the criteria desired. The nursing unit form can be characterized by the type of circulation patterns, such as single corridor, double corridor, the cluster, and work corridor. In addition, there are many variations and combinations of each plan type.

#### SINGLE CORRIDOR PLAN

The oldest hospital plan form was the open ward. The single corridor plan resulted from enclosing the bed areas into separate roms. Prior to air conditioning and artificial ventilation, all rooms required outside windows. Generally, the single corridor plan locates rooms on either side of the corridor, with the nursing station at the center of the unit. The greatest weakness of this plan lies in the extreme corridor length required for nursing units of any appreciable size. As hospitals developed, the lengths of corridors became so great that it was necessary to limit their distance by law. Hospital regulations specified that the distance between a nursing station and the furthest bedroom door should not exceed ninety feet.

Most single corridor plans negate the very qualities desired for children. Hallways are long and frightening; the nurse has no direct visual supervision over children except for the few she can see from the nurse's station; and if the nurse's station is located in the center of the unit, control of the entrances is difficult.

A notable exception to the standard single corridor plan is one designed as a prototype for the Nuffield Foundation (see Plan I). The corridor is shortened and widened to make it partially a work corridor. A large ward opens directly on the corridor, which turns the area into a light and pleasant place. The careful thought given to mothers' accommodations, joint use of facilities by several units, direct and easy access to the out-of-doors, and the well-controlled entrances and exits make it a cheerful, workable environment for pediatric patients.

## Plan 1. Modified Single Corridor

**Model Children's Ward**

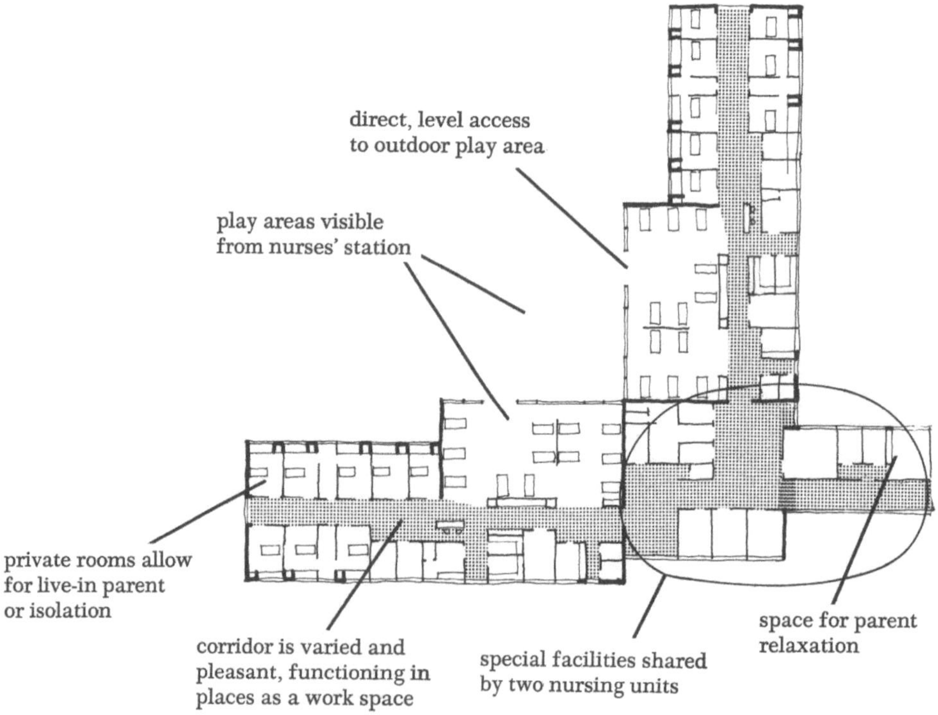

DOUBLE CORRIDOR PLAN

The most typical plan type used since World War II is the double corridor, which was created in an effort simultaneously to increase the size of the unit, to centralize the service and transportation facilities, and to cut down the length of the corridor. Generally speaking, the double corridor plan locates the beds on the periphery and the nursing station, treatment rooms, utility rooms, transportation facilities, and offices in an artificially ventilated or air-conditioned interior core. Periodically placed secondary corridors link both sides of the unit together.

As nursing unit sizes increased, difficulties arose with the double corridor plan. The distances became greater, the hallways longer, and the visibility less. More persons were required to service the unit, and inevitably the patient felt more and more like a cog in an institutional machine. Although this is not a good plan type for pediatric use, many pediatric departments were forced into this mold because of restrictions of the overall hospital layout and design. The double corridor becomes more workable for pediatric use when subdivided into sections having a separate nursing station in each section, a revision that allows for both the separation of age groups and contact between them.

The Pediatric Unit of the Colorado General Hospital in Denver has a dougle corridor plan (see Plan 2). The west wing, which was built as one nursing unit, is now functionally two: one unit for children from three to ten, the other for preteens and teens. The east wing has always been separated into two, with one unit for premature newborns and another for infants and toddlers. Within each unit are substations that bring the nurse closer to the child. The best feature of these units is the availability of very large roof decks on the same level. When developed with adequate soft surfacing, planting, and play materials, these decks will provide a range of freedom and experience seldom available to the child hospitalized in an urban setting.

Wyler's Children Hospital in Chicago, the Children's Hospital of Los Angeles, and Worcester City Hospital, Massachusetts, have double corridor plans (see Plans 3–5). Their greatest problems are lack of direct visual supervision, the long corridors, and the difficulty in controlling entrance and exits. On the positive side is the easy access to treatment facilities, the centralization of services, and particularly in Children's Hospital and the Colorado General Hospital, the subdivision of the unit into different age groups. Both the Colorado General Hospital and the Children's Medical and Surgical Center of Johns Hopkins Hospital, Baltimore, have adjacent doctors' research facilities and laboratories, which have allowed a fruitful dialogue between students, resident staff, and faculty.

## Plan 2. Double Corridor

Colorado General Hospital,
Denver, Colorado

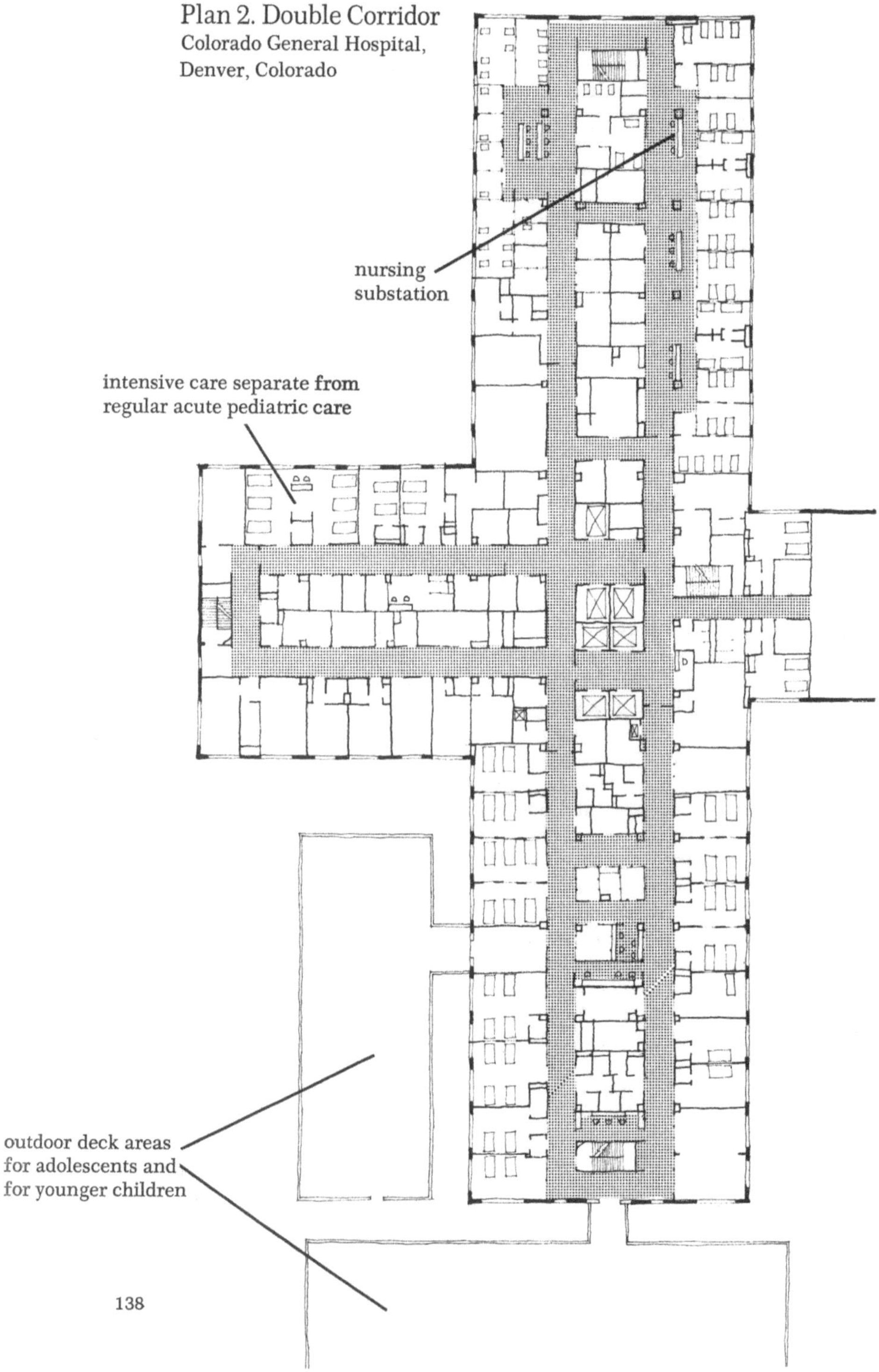

## Plan 3. Double Corridor with Adjoining Research Wing

**Wyler Children's Hospital, Chicago, Illinois**

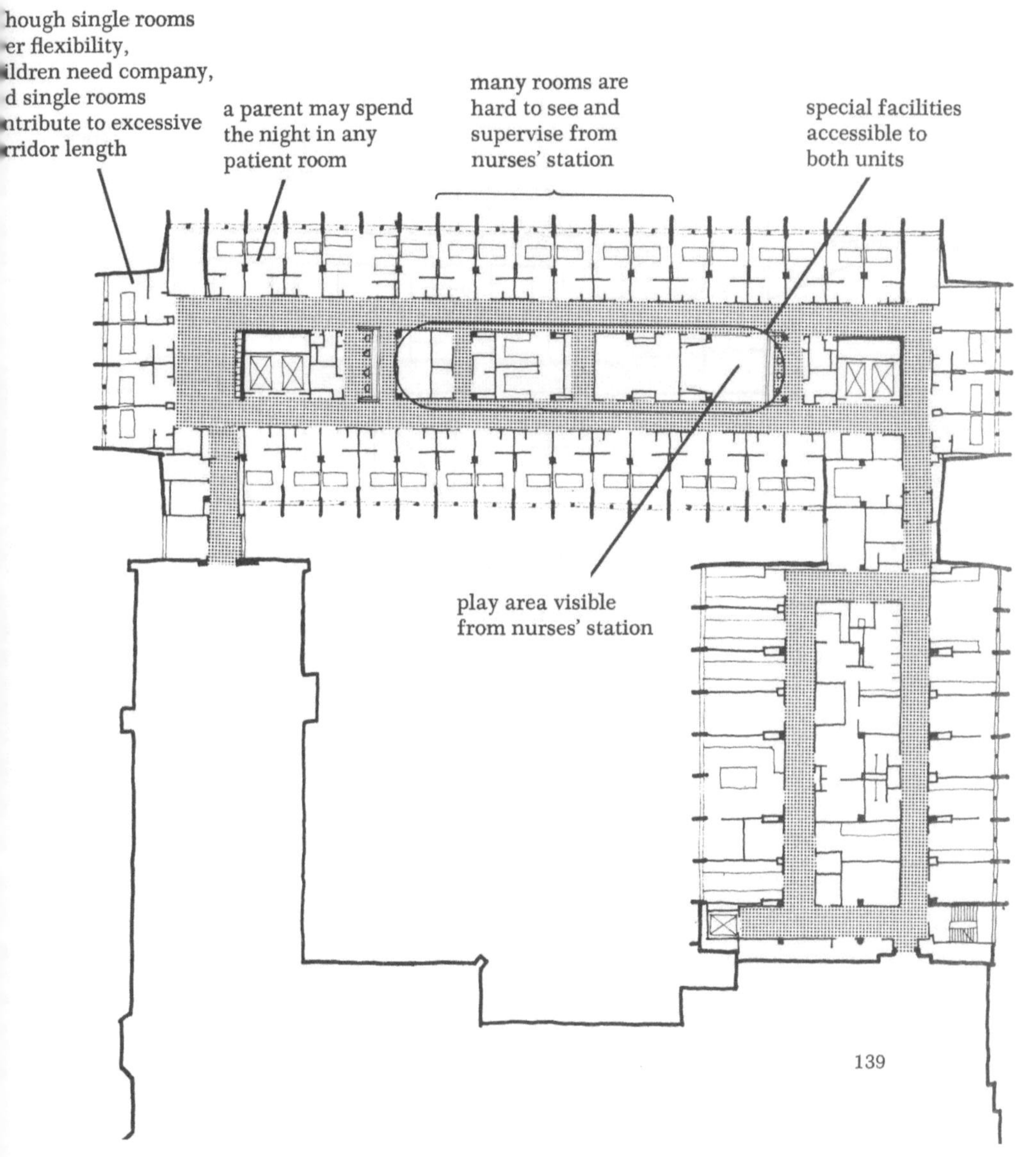

## Plan 4. Double Corridor
### Adolescent Unit, Children's Hospital of Los Angeles

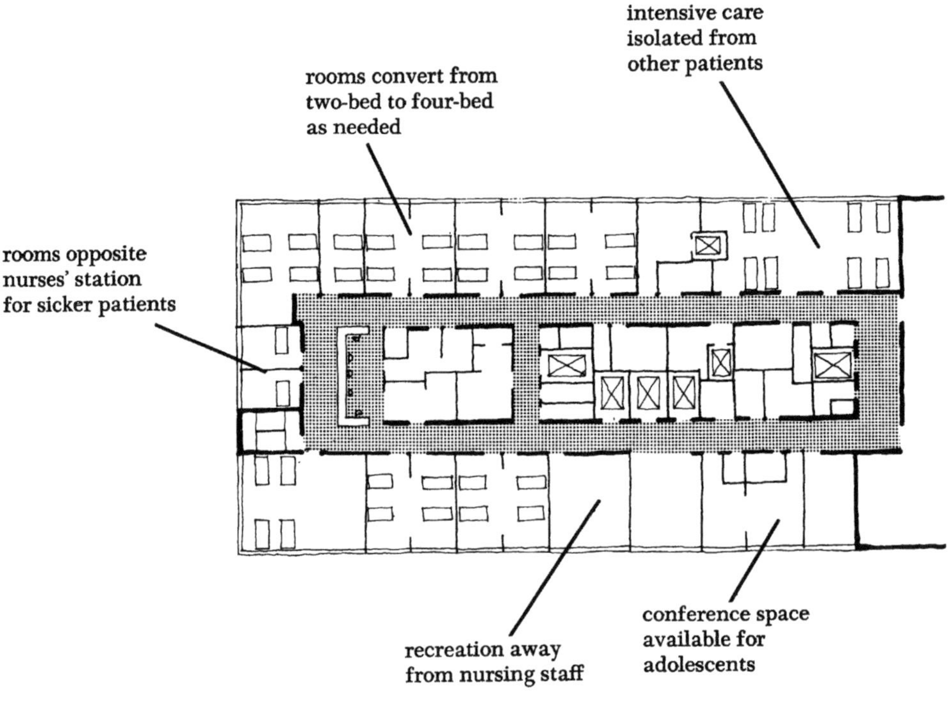

## Plan 5. Modified Double Corridor

**Worcester City Hospital, Worcester, Massachusetts**

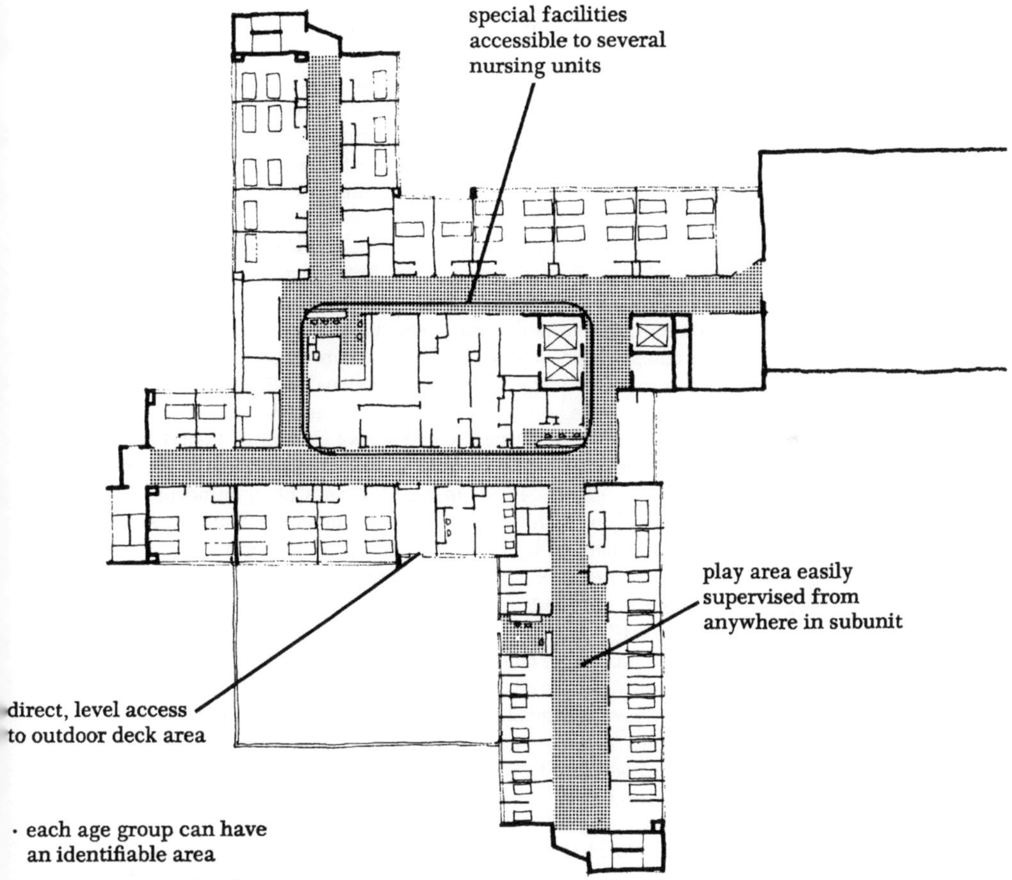


- each age group can have an identifiable area
- units can expand and contract as needed

THE CLUSTER

The most recent basic form for the nursing unit returns to some of the characteristics of the original open ward system — a central space around which are clustered other areas. This cluster may be circular, square, or highly irregular and still retain the same compact topology.

The compact nature of the cluster has many advantages for pediatric use. It affords visibility from a central place and eliminates long corridors. Even when in bed, children can see the nurses' work area and feel that they are being cared for. Clusters can have a residential scale and feeling that encourages close personal contact between patients and staff and creates a sense of place, providing the child with an identifiable home unit within the hospital.

The close proximity of the nurse to the patient is predicated on a system of delivery of supplies, transporting laundry, food, medications, and other needed supplies to the nurse instead of requiring the nurse to travel to a central source to obtain them. Some plans are being developed which in effect extend this concept of operation and eliminate the nurses' station entirely. Instead of a nurses' station, each bedroom contains space for charting, pneumatic tubes, supplies, medication, and disposal.

Children's Hospital at Stanford consists of four clustered nursing units. Each cluster is self-contained for a certain age group and is an architecturally independent, identifiable unit (see Plan 6). The division into three, and ultimately four, age groupings has provided possibilities for many excellent programs. The unusually spacious design makes it possible for children in beds, on gurneys, and in wheelchairs to leave the bedrooms and take part in play therapy and school programs. Visual access to the landscaped grounds is pleasant and pervasive. Access to the outdoors is potentially excellent. The younger children's playground provides opportunities for children with various degrees of mobility. The tree house, for example, can be reached by rope, ladder, stairs, or ramp. At present, however, parents are not specially provided for. A care-by-parent unit in a separate building is planned.

St. Luke's Hospital in St. Paul, Minnesota, Mercy Hospital in Redding, California, and the protypical college health center plan of the Educational Facilities Laboratories use the circular cluster (see Plans 7–8). In each case the configuration allows for good visual contact between nursing staff and patients at all times. Offices, examination space, bathrooms, and other spaces requiring privacy are located on the periphery of the nursing units to allow an unobstructed visual field. At St. Luke's, three clusters jointly use a core of enclosed specialized facilities.

Lincoln General Hospital in Lincoln, Nebraska, provides an example of a basically identical configuration achieved with a rectangular building system (see Plan 9). Particularly interesting is the psychiatric unit, which demonstrates the use of an off-center nursing station — appropriate to units requiring less intense visual supervision, such as psychiatric or convalescent adolescent units.

The Boston Floating Hospital proposal demonstrated the use of small ten-bed clusters within the large building necessary in an urban medical center (see Plan 10). Within this framework, each unit is provided with some sense of identity and direct access to an outdoor area. Specialized facilities are conveniently located near each unit.

Two other approaches to the problem of organizing clusters within a large hospital are provided by the TOAM entry in an Israeli architectural competition and a proposal for the Pacific Medical Center in San Francisco (see Plans 11–12). The Israeli example uses, in effect, clusters of clusters. Four eight-bed wards open onto both a large nursing work area and day room and an outdoor deck area. This hierarchical development of space has resulted in a particularly clear and direct circulation system.

In the Pacific Medical Center project the architects have created a continuous, overlapping system of clusters. The overlapping areas between clusters make it possible for units to expand and contract as needed. The location of nursing stations allows two or three units to be supervised from one station when necessary, as at night.

## Plan 6. Cluster Units off Double Corridor Core

Children's Hospital at Stanford, Palo Alto, California

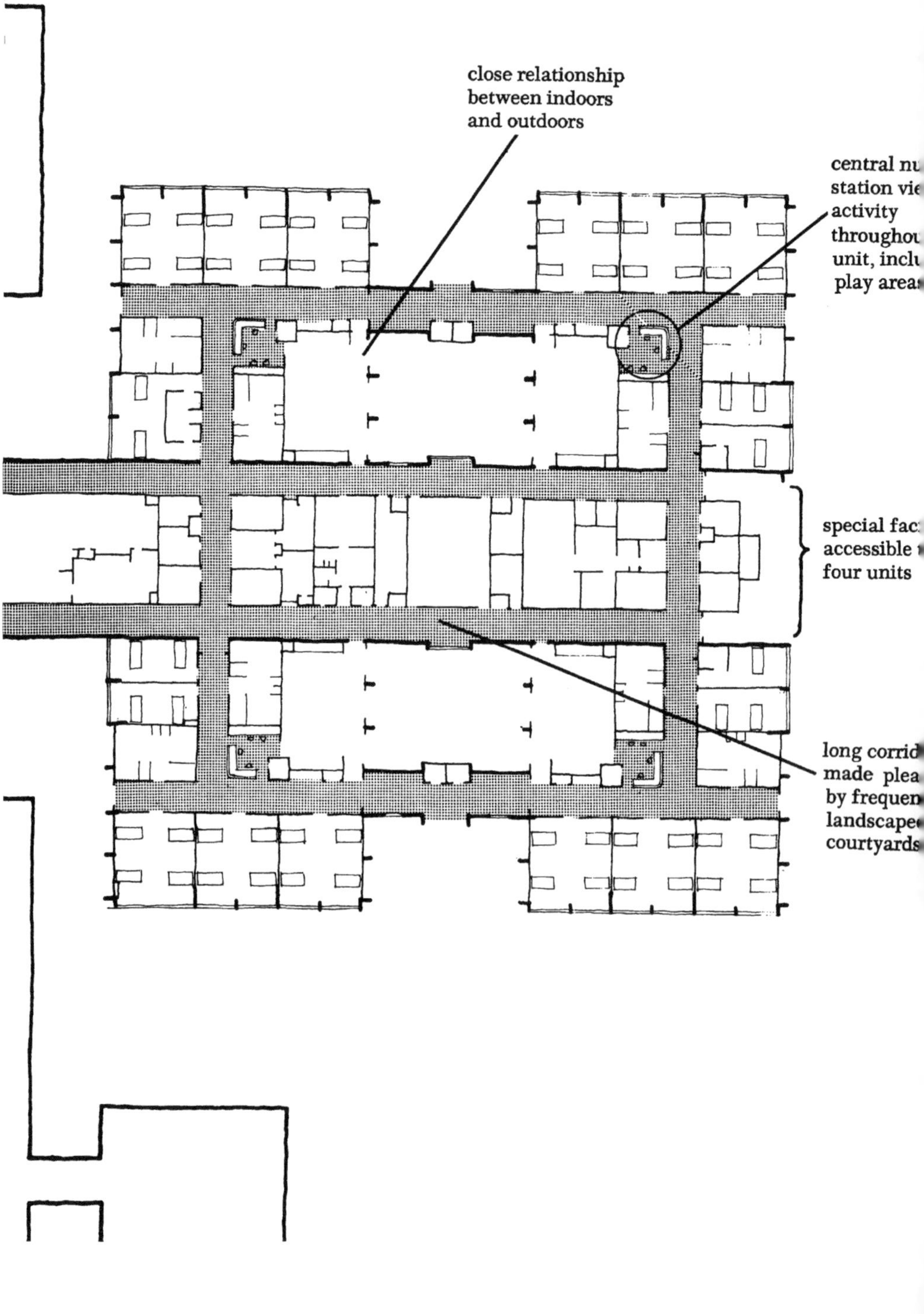

## Plan 7. Grouped Circular Clusters
**St. Luke's Hospital, St. Paul, Minnesota**

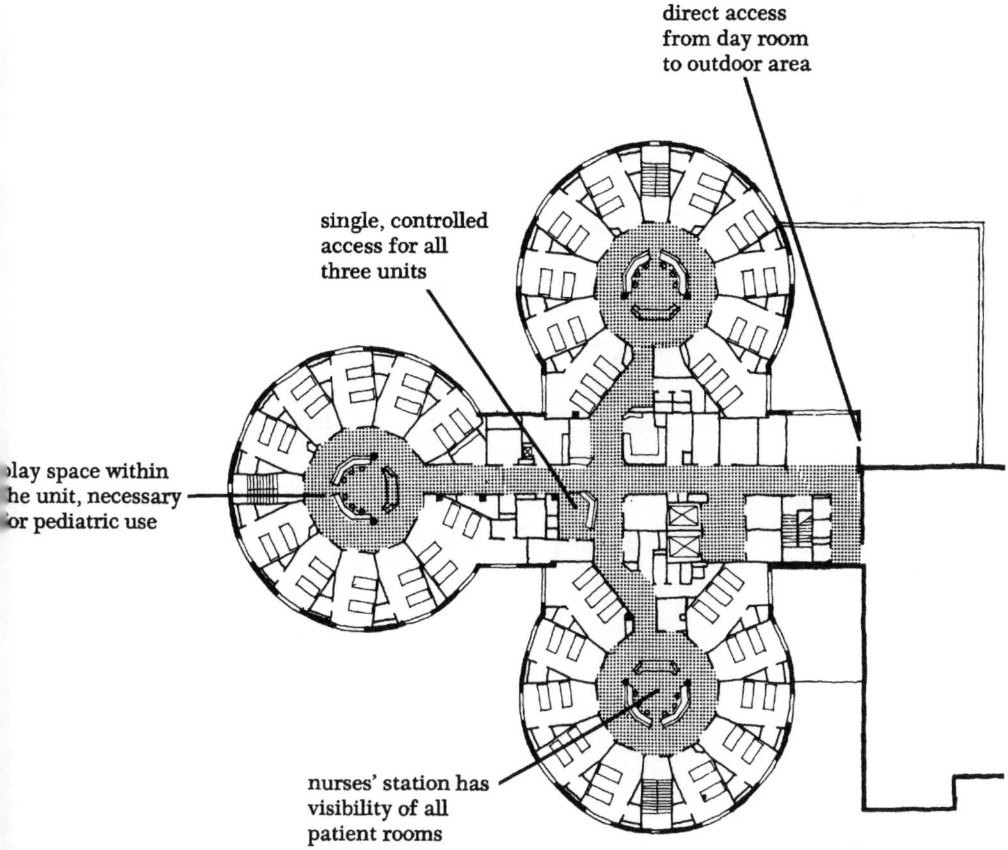

## Plan 8. Circular Cluster

**Above: Protypical College Health Center**
**Below: Pediatrics Pavilion, Mercy Hospital, Redding, California**

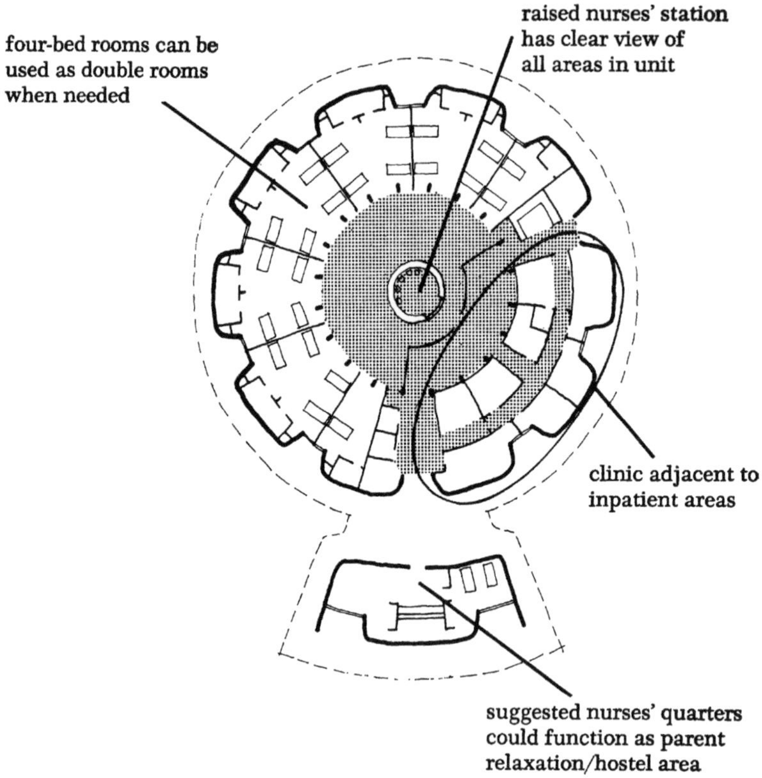


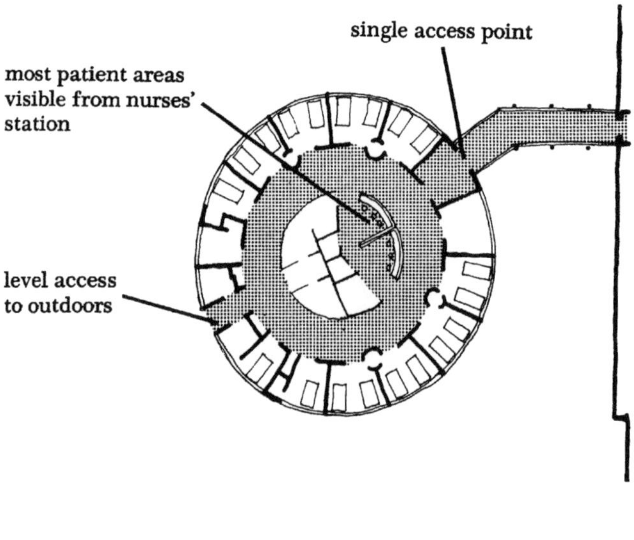

# Plan 9. Grouped Rectilinear Clusters

Lincoln General Hospital, Lincoln, Nebraska

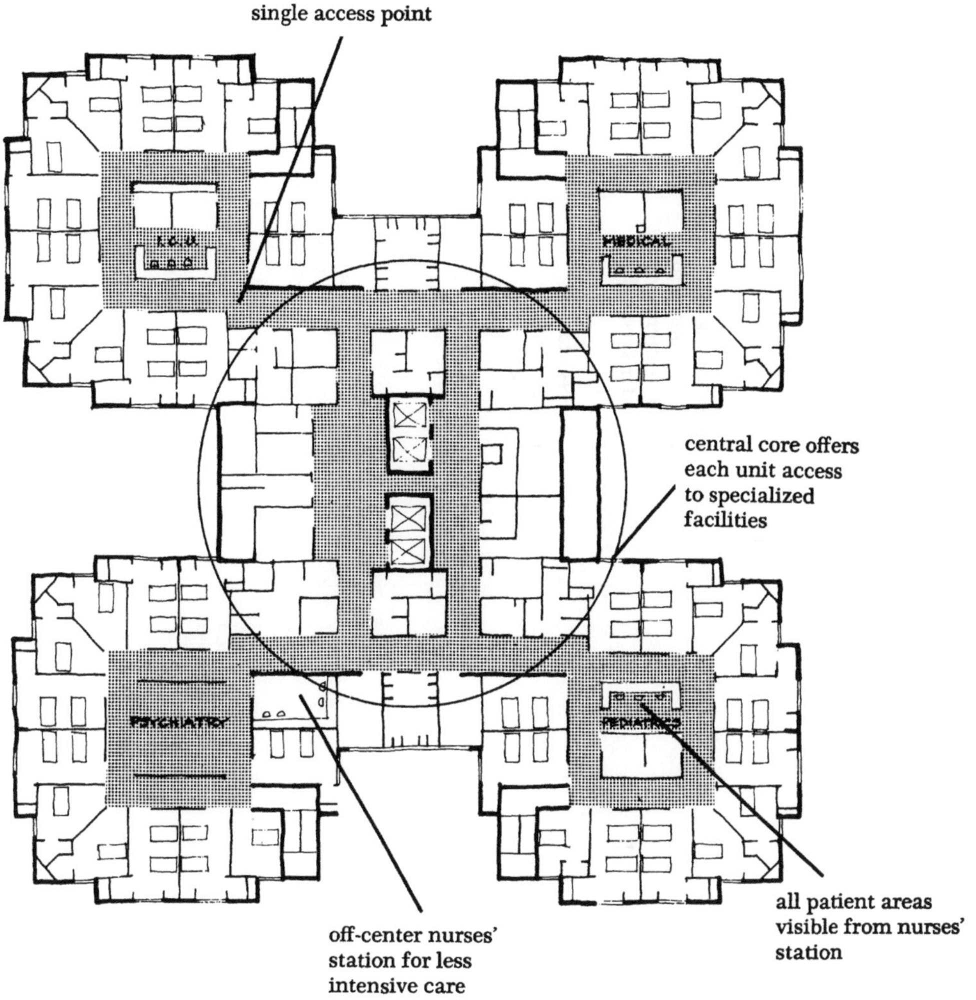

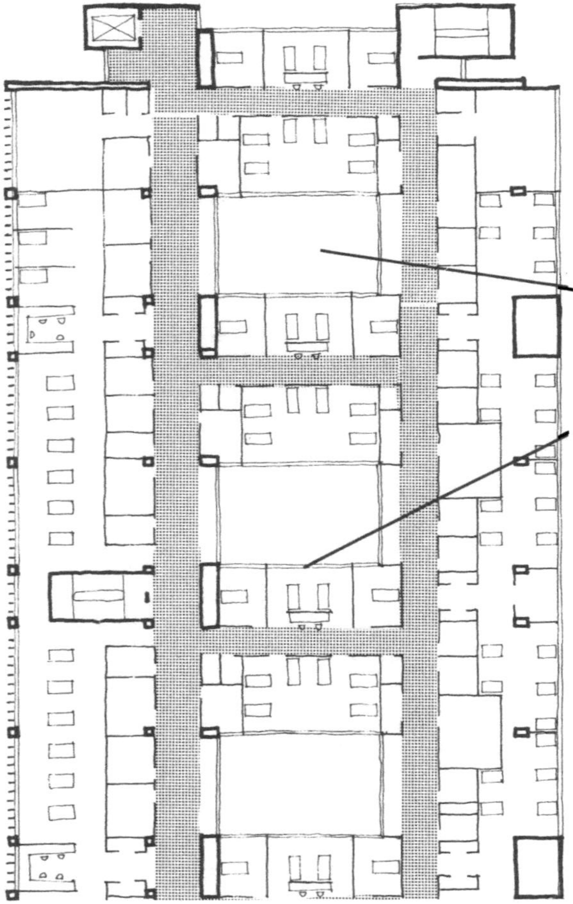

visual access to
pleasant courtyards
makes extremely long
corridor acceptable

direct access to
courtyards for
many units

- provision for parents
to live in on
another floor

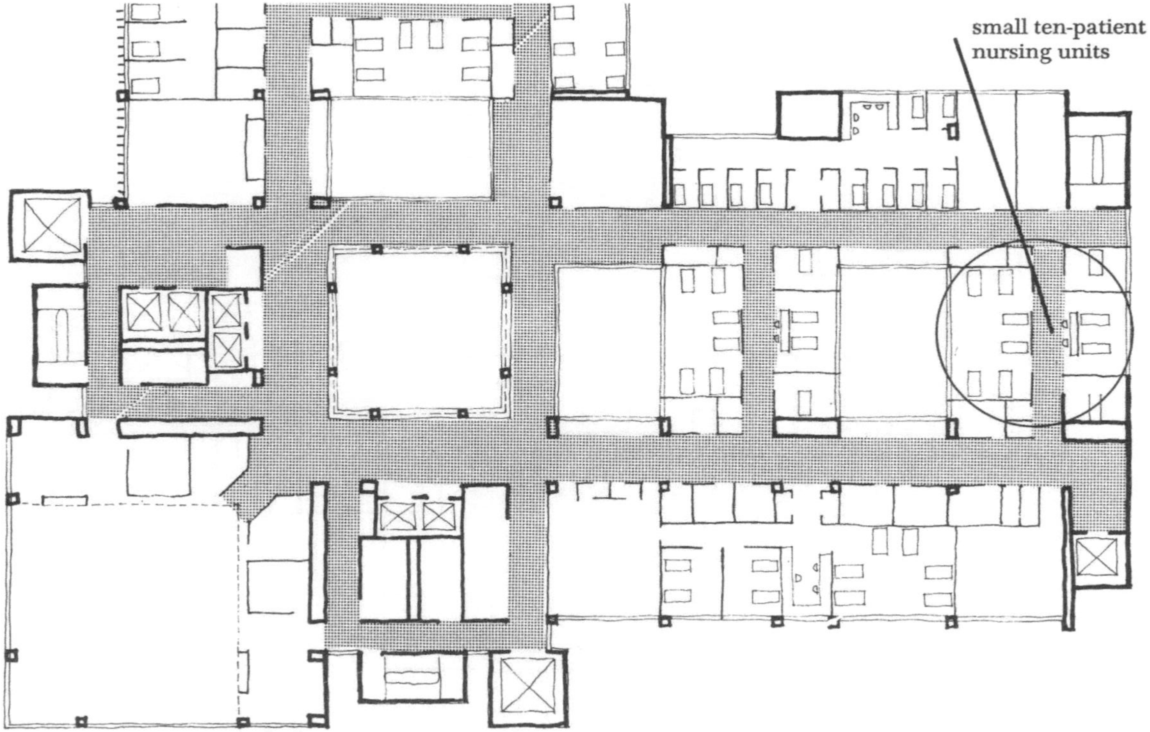


Plan 10. Grouped Rectangular Clusters
**Proposal for Boston Floating Hospital, Tufts-New England Medical Center**

## Plan 11. Grouped Rectangular Clusters

**Entry in Architectural Competition, Israel**

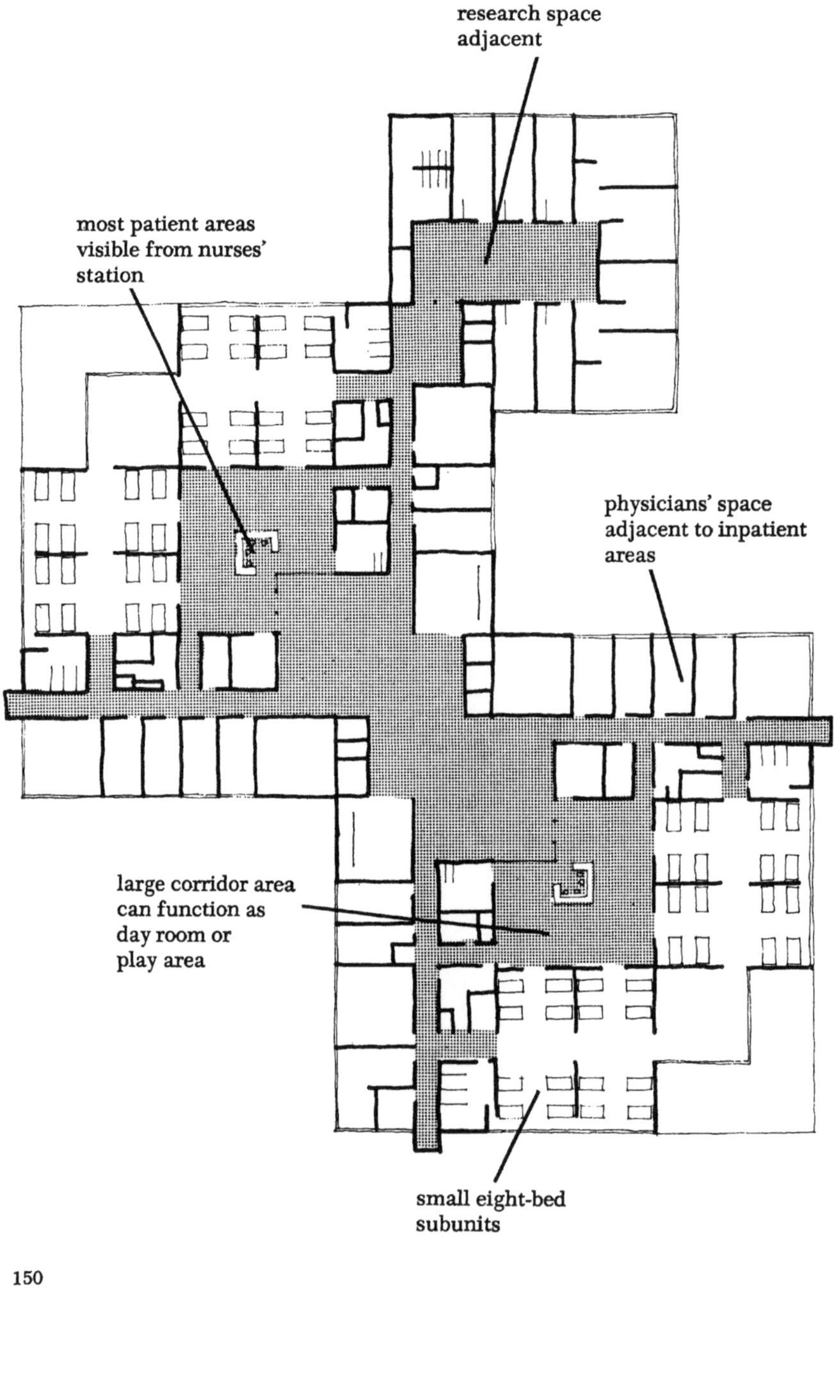

## Plan 12. Continuous Overlapping Clusters
Proposal for Pacific Medical Center, San Francisco, California

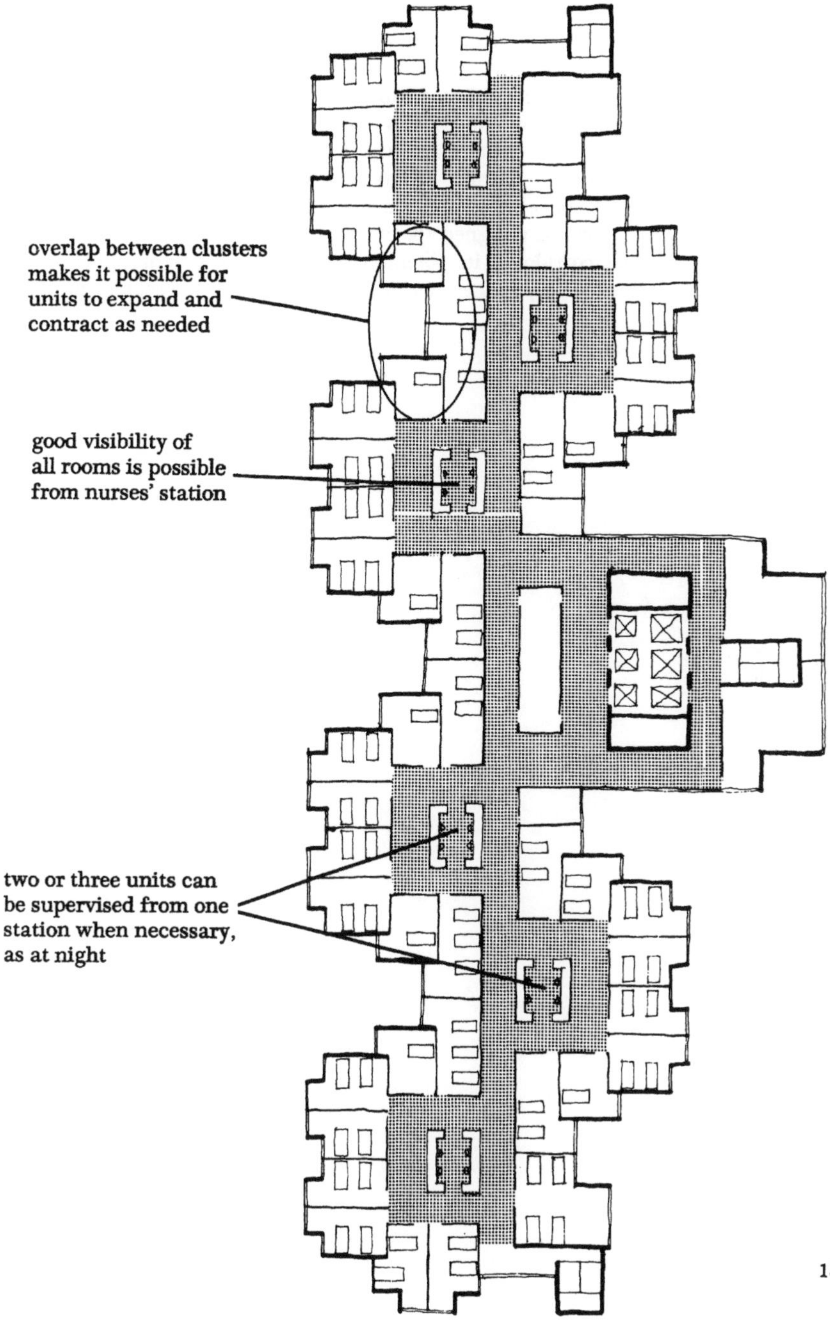

THE WORK CORRIDOR PLAN

The work corridor, a plan form developed by the Kaiser Foundation, uses the central corridor area as both a work place and a circulation space for patients and staff. A secondary traffic route developed around the outside accommodates visitors. This idea has been used with the organization of the nursing unit into smaller clusters servicing from eight to twelve patients.

The Kaiser Foundation Hospitals in Santa Clara and Panorama City, California, show two uses of the work corridor (see Plan 13). In Santa Clara, nursing clusters are strung along the work corridor with a visitor's corridor on the outside. At Panorama City the clusters group around a central work space with visitors again using an outside corridor. Neither of the units shown is designed specifically for pediatric use. An advantage of the exterior corridor is its potential as a place for parents quite separate and complementary to the interior work corridor for the regular nursing staff.

Plan 13. Work Corridor
Kaiser Foundation Hospitals
Above: Santa Clara, California
Below: Panorama City, California

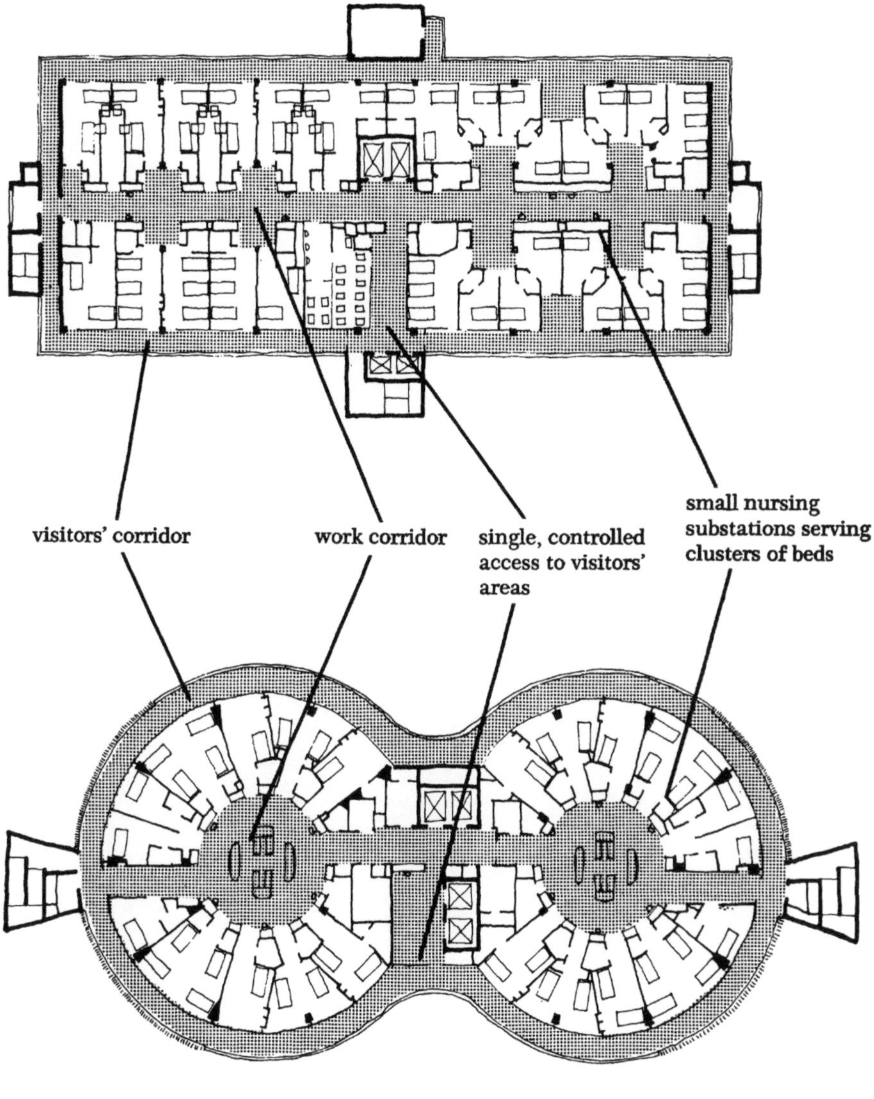

# Appendix A Design Guidelines for Evaluating Pediatric Nursing Units

Every projected building plan must be looked at in the context of the total health care system to determine whether it implements the desired medical and social program. To this end, a checklist is provided for use as an evaluative tool.

## Alternatives to Hospitalization

Are preventive, diagnostic, therapeutic, and rehabilitative facilities available for all in the community regardless of income, ethnic group, social status, or vocation?

— neighborhood health stations
— babysitting service
— separate facilities for teenagers
— school clinics
— school infirmaries
— preventive medicine/recreation centers
— health jitneys
— mobile health units
— other facilities
—

Are facilities and programs available for partial hospitalization?

— day hospitals
— night hospitals
— bus and ambulance service for non-acutely ill patients
— aided home care programs
— housekeeping services
— home remodeling services for handicapped
— communications links among home, hospital, and school
— other facilities and programs
—

## The Hospital Environment and the Community

Are all potential hospital users represented on decision-making bodies involved in planning programs and facilities?

— members of all subgroups in the community — racial, ethnic, economic, or otherwise, particularly parents and children
— members of all job categories in the hospital, professional or nonprofessional
— students planning health careers
— volunteer workers in the hospital
— other users
—

Have health workers and community members been given adequate instruction in understanding physical plans?

— visual aids
— relating scale drawings to built forms in visits to existing facilities
— other instruction
—

Does the hospital environment present an accessible and reassuring image to the community?

Entry:

— pleasant, direct path between outside transportation (car, bus, taxi, ambulance) and pediatric unit
— separate pediatric entrance to hospital
— separate pediatric emergency entrance and waiting area
— admittance by nursing staff from nursing unit
— other features
—

Circulation and Waiting:

— clear and short circulation patterns
— pleasant corridors with diffuse lighting, outside views, special alcoves for waiting
— waiting areas with diverting things to do
— storage and equipment space out of view
— other features
—

## The Overall Nursing Environment

Are appropriate facilities available for all users of the pediatric nursing environment?

— infants
— young children
— grade school children
— adolescents
— mothers

— fathers
— siblings
— nursing staff, including registered nurses, aides, licensed vocational nurses
— physicians
— students
— social service workers
— technicians and therapists
— the staff as a team
— other users
—

Are nursing units (or subunits) small enough to encourage close personal relations?

— subunits of 3–5 infants
— units of 6–8 young children
— units of 12–16 grade school children
— units of 8–24 adolescents
— units of about 8 children with parents for care-by-parent
— other
—

Is there adequate communication and interaction between units for children of different ages?

— shared facilities
— permeable boundaries
— other opportunities for interaction
—

Are specialized facilities easily accessible to the nursing units?

— family space
— student areas
— nurses' space
— doctors' examination and treatment areas
— team space
— demonstration room
— other offices
— diagnostic, treatment, and consultation facilities accessible to both ambulant and bed patients
—

Does each pediatric unit have direct access to the outside?

— ground area
— roof deck
— no level changes between indoor and outdoor areas

— shade structures, wind screening where necessary to increase outdoor season
— surfaces appropriate for walking, playing, and other activities for persons in wheelchairs, on crutches, on gurneys, or in beds
— other facilities for outdoor use
—

Does the design of each unit provide for the possibility of variations in size and use?

— overlap between units or subunits to allow increases or decreases in size
— scale suitable for younger or older children and adults
— single bedrooms convertible to doubles
— double bedrooms convertible to four-bed wards
— walls that can be transparent or opaque
— adaptable multipurpose space for each unit consisting of a central space with two or more subspaces
— movable furniture
— other features allowing flexible use
—

## Environments for Infants (0–12 Months)

Does the environment encourage a close, mothering relationship with each infant?

— small unit size
— self-contained subunits
— convenient, close-by services
— comfortable feeding areas
— privacy for breast feeding
— facilities that encourage parent participation
— other facilities encouraging close, warm relations between infants and caretakers
—

Does the environment include safe, pleasant places for infants to develop motor skills?

— indoor crawling area or a "giant playpen" with a warm, soft floor
— outdoor crawling area with soft surfacing
— no electrical outlets, chemicals, or sharp or hot objects below forty inches
— other opportunities to develop motor skills
—

Does the environment provide stimulating sensory experiences for infants?

— movement, especially human activity, visible from crib
— natural lighting in all spaces used by infants
— patterned and textured materials for curtains, walls, floors
— music
— other stimulation
—

## Environments for Toddlers (1–3 Years) and Preschoolers (3–6 Years)

Does the environment allow direct visual supervision of young children at all times?

— unobstructed visual field from nurses' station to all indoor and outdoor patient areas within the nursing unit
— glazed partitions
— other techniques for visual supervision
—

Is the environment safe for young children?

— single, well-controlled entrance to unit
— low beds or cribs
— no oxygen outlets, electrical outlets, hot or sharp objects, or other potentially dangerous objects below fifty-five inches
— all glazed areas made of tempered glass or unbreakable plastic
— glazed doors
— medication preparation area well-equipped, quiet, and lockable
— other safety features
—

Can the young child keep in touch with his family?

— available telephones
— windows overlooking streets and parking area used by visiting parents and linking the child with the outside
— facilities for parent to live in and stay overnight
— other ways to maintain contact
—

Is the scale of the environment appropriate for both young children and adults?

— small groupings of a social scale comprehensible to young children
— raised facilities for eating, playing, and bathing so that an adult can help a child without bending
— variations in ceiling heights and changes in levels to allow a child to feel big and an adult to look small by contrast

— adjustable height beds and cribs — low for children, high for nurses when working
— generally high ceiling height to minimize adults' heights, with very low ceiling height alcoves for children's play
— opportunities for safe climbing
— low window sills
— low sinks and toilets
— low mirrors
— low hanging rods for clothing
— warm, easily cleaned floors
— good lighting at floor level for drawing and other close work
— other features convenient to both adults and children
—

Does the environment encourage young children to care for themselves when possible?

— easily cleaned eating areas for small groups of young children
— feeding tables or highchairs for toddlers
— low washbasins with clearance beneath for juvenile wheelchairs
— private storage place for clothing and belongings at child's level
— visible toilets accessible to all play areas, indoors and out
— potty chairs for toddlers
— open toilets supervisable by nurse at distance
— other provisions for self-care
—

Does the environment offer adequate challenge and stimulation for young children?

— indoor and outdoor play areas accessible and easily supervised from nurses' work area
— storage indoors and out for a rich variety of play materials
— opportunities for water play indoors and out
— baths
— raised water areas for water play for children in gurneys and wheelchairs
— well-equipped areas for crafts, blocks, messy play
— a variety of interior floor surfaces, for sitting or napping, messy activities, wheeled toys
— outdoor play area directly accessible and supervisable from indoor play area
— a variety of outdoor surfaces, for wheeled toys, digging, water play, under playground equipment
—growing plants and animals to care for and observe
— other challenges
—

## Environments for Grade School Children (6–12 Years)

Does the environment provide opportunities for grade school children to continue to acquire and exercise cognitive and motor skills?

— hospital classroom, large enough to accommodate beds or gurneys
— classroom outside medical environment
— electronic links to home schools
— classroom aides for use by the weak or handicapped
— soundproofed music practice room
— large outdoor play area
— athletic opportunities for all children, even those whose physical activity is limited
— settings for imaginative outdoor play: planting, play sheds
— materials for construction of clubhouses and other enclosed places
— other opportunities for skills development
—

Does the environment encourage the ability of grade school children to live and work with others?

— shared bedrooms for about four same-sex children
— project space near each bed
— large, multipurpose group dining area
— subdivision of multipurpose area possible
— generous storage for craft materials, tools, table games, books in multipurpose area
— kitchenette for snacks, bag lunches, cooking projects
— other opportunities for group contact
—

Are there opportunities for grade school children to assume responsibility?

— special devices necessary for independent toileting and washing of disabled and weak children
— private storage space for personal belongings, projects, and clothing
— nonallergenic animals and plants for children to care for
— other opportunities for self-care and care of others
—

## Environments for Adolescents (12–18 Years)

Is the adolescent provided with opportunities to develop a sense of his own identity?

— a choice of room accommodations: one, two, and four-bed rooms
— a personal space for each patient, large enough for medical equipment, personal possessions, and visitors

— opportunities to decorate and personalize this space
— privacy when needed or wanted in personal space
— a window in each personal space
— no direct surveillance of personal space from nurses' station, but casual surveillance of all bed spaces possible from hallway
— a quiet, pleasant room with complete privacy available for conversation, meditation
— other facilities for expressing and developing identity
—

Does the environment allow the adolescent to maintain a positive body image?

— bathrooms isolated from living spaces to ensure acoustic and olfactory privacy
— bathtub room separate from, but adjacent to, toilet and lavatory
— no gang bathrooms
— bathrooms easily used without aid by the weak or disabled
— bathrooms large enough for use with attendant if necessary
— attractive bathroom areas for grooming and self-care
— clothing care facilities: washer, dryer, iron and ironing board, sewing machine
— facilities for exercise and athletics
— other facilities for maintaining a body image
—

Does the environment allow opportunities for adolescents to exercise individual independence and responsibility?

— teen sanctuary where adolescent activity can occur free from close supervision without disturbing sicker patients
— movable, changeable furnishings and decorations in teen sanctuary
— comfortable floor for sitting
— snack bar
— separate teen day room for studying, TV, and dining
— day room large enough to accommodate several small tables
— variable lighting levels in teen room
— subspaces off teen day room for individual activities
— kitchenette adjacent to teen day room
— telephone jacks near every bed
— large, private telephone alcove for gurneys and wheelchairs
— other opportunities for independence
—

Does the environment provide opportunities for adolescents' cognitive development?

— schoolroom
— electronic links to home schools

— electronic learning environment
— other forms
—

## Environments for Family Participation

Are services and facilities available to enable parents to be with their sick children?

— hospital jitney service
— sibling child care facility at or near the hospital
— inexpensive parents' accommodations near hospital
— inexpensive meal service for parents
— other services and facilities
—

Does the environment provide a range of opportunities for parents to care for their children?

Overnight Accommodations:

— private rooms with baths on each nursing unit to accommodate parents overnight
— storage space for visiting parents' possessions
— other facilities
—

Parents' Station:

— territory to store equipment and to work without interfering with nurses' domain
— food preparation area for parent use
— other facilities
—

Are there places in the environment for parents to rest and relax away from their children?

— pleasant, residential parent lounge
— snack bar
— quiet area with comfortable bed for napping
— toilet and shower facilities for both mothers and fathers
— visual distraction: interesting views, textured and patterned materials
— other provisions
—

Does the environment provide for the option of care-by-parent?

— separate room that can function as a living room as well as a bedroom and bath for each parent and patient

— accommodations for siblings
— family-like lounge for socializing, preparation of snacks
— laundry and storage for not more than eight patients and families
— immediate access to professional nurses, staff physicians, and special equipment for medical emergencies
— opportunities for meaningful work and learning activities for parents
— other opportunities for parent care
—

## Environments for Staff

Does the environment encourage staff communication and teamwork?

— pleasant, informal meeting place for six to twelve people near pediatric unit
— round table, comfortable chairs, coffee pot
— teaching aids, blackboards, tackboards
— sound isolated from patient area
— other facilities for staff interaction
—

Does the environment encourage community participation on the health team?

— programs to involve every subgroup in the community, especially minorities and men
— teaching and volunteer space for these programs
— other means for community involvement
—

Does the environment provide nurses with opportunities for close patient contact and job satisfaction?

— a territory and personal space for each member of the nursing staff
— direct visual contact with children
— nurses' substation for "bedside nurse" and aide responsible for from four to eight patients
— work and storage space at each substation
— specialized facilities for medication preparation, storage of drugs
— a flexible record and communication system designed to allow supervision of several substations from one place at night or off-hours
— informal consultation space
— lounge and locker space away from pediatric unit
— other facilities
—

Does the environment encourage students' and physicians' concern for patients as individuals while providing opportunities for observation and consultation?

Alternatives to Medical Rounds:

— closed circuit TV system at each patient's bed
— closed circuit TV system in examination-treatment spaces
— TV viewing rooms for staff and students
— demonstration room with large, raised observation area behind one-way mirrors
— other alternatives
—

Other Facilities:

— additional space allowed throughout unit for students for charting, medicine preparation, treatments
— small student-faculty meeting rooms near pediatric unit
— other facilities enabling students to learn without disturbing patients
—

Does the environment allow physicians to work quickly and efficiently without sacrificing the social and emotional needs of the pediatric patient?

— sufficient numbers of examination-treatment and consultation rooms to minimize time spent by doctors waiting for patients
— dictation equipment, x-ray viewing, desk space available to each physician
— privacy and informality in examination and treatment space
— consultation space easily accessible from corridor
— visual aides available for explaining diseases to patients
— other facilities for physicians
—

# Appendix B
# Observations of Children in Hospitals

A series of observations was carried on over a period of several months in six hospitals that were considered to offer a high level of patient care. Statistical material was not collected; rather, a subjective evaluation of the individual children's reactions to the hospital was attempted. The three observations reported here give not only an objective picture of what happened to specific children on certain typical days in different community hospitals, but also indicate some of the programmatic and architectural implications of these occurrences. These observations were made over a series of several days in April 1970 by Christie Coffin and Jacqueline Vischer.

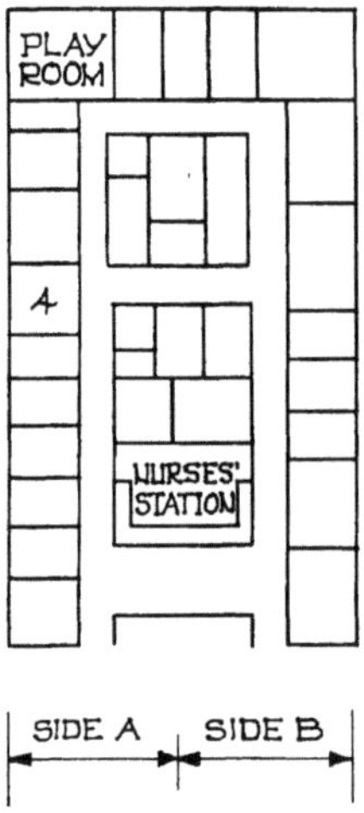


## Infants and Young Children

Five patients in one room, aged three months to five years, were observed for eighteen hours over two days.

Location: a community hospital, Pediatrics Unit, Side A, for fifteen–twenty children from birth to 6 years old. Room 4, a five-bed room used for children not requiring isolation or intensive nursing care.

PERSONAE

*Alice* (3 months), a patient who has been in the hospital five days with severe bronchitis. She is in a mist tent.

*Brenda* (21 months), a patient recovering from meningitis, which has kept her in the hospital for several weeks.

*Colin* (3 years), a patient with a bone disease affecting

one knee, who has been in the hospital for nine days. He was hospitalized once before at age two.

*Douglas* (3 1/2 years), a patient who was operated on the day before for a hand deformity.

*Earl* (5 years), a patient who has been hospitalized several days and is nearly recovered except for a cough and fluctuating fever.

Nursing staff: RN *Allen*, RN *Benson*, and three others who appear briefly and are not named.

Medical staff: three outside physicians, two interns, and one resident.

Visitors: Alice's mother, Colin's mother.

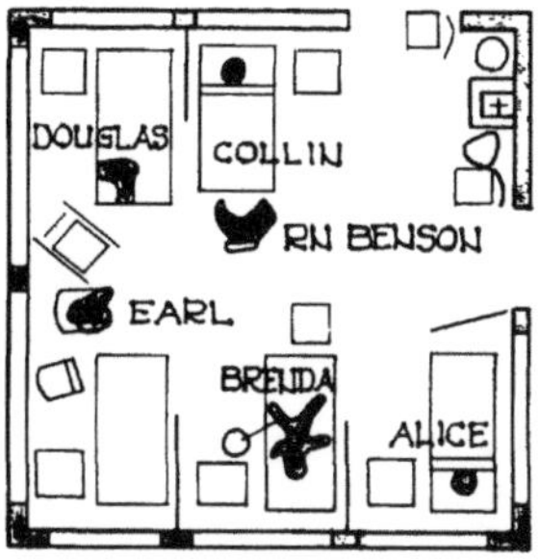


*9:30* Colin is wheeled out into the hallway in his wheelchair. He is left sitting in front of the nurses' station near a large fish bowl.

Earl is in the rocking chair playing quietly.

Douglas is walking up and down in bed. The nurse continually reminds him to keep his arm with the cast on it above his heart so that it won't hurt.

Brenda, having just displaced an IV needle in transit from another part of the hospital, is in her bed fighting an intern, a resident, and RN Benson, who are attempting to insert another IV needle. She is purple with rage. When the IV needle is finally inserted, the resident and RN Benson attach restraints to her arms and legs. Tired from her struggle, she soon falls asleep. [It is not convenient to use the children's beds to transport them through the corridors; gurneys, being slimmer, are more easily maneuvered in the limited space. However, space to maneuver beds through doors and corridors might have prevented this scene.]

Alice cannot be seen in her mist tent, which provides an opaque fog.

RN Benson works briskly, going from child to child, bathing them and changing their clothing.

*10:00* Douglas is very impatient, walking all over in his bed. "Me next, me next," he says as RN Benson goes about her duties. [The playroom cannot be supervised from Rooms 4 and 5 or from the nurses' work area, making it necessary to keep children in bed unless a supervisor is available for the playroom.]

Douglas watches television while RN Benson readies the other children for the day. The television program, giving advice on filling out income tax returns, does not hold his attention for long.

Alice's mother comes in and sits in the baby's cubicle. She looks into the mists for some time. The baby is still not visible. [The small cubicles allotted each child and parent give them a territory in which they can feel more at home. Unfortunately shared territory in which they might be encouraged to have useful contact with others is missing.]

The intern comes in to look at Alice, takes her out of the mist tent, looks at her, and chats with her mother.

*10:10* Earl continues to play in the rocking chair; Douglas hums little tunes and walks up and down in his bed, and RN Benson scolds him for forgetting to keep his arm up. Brenda sleeps. An occupational therapist and a volunteer come in to say hello to Earl and go out. RN Allen comes in to help Douglas out of bed.

*10:25* Earl and Douglas leave with the therapist and volunteer. RN Allen makes Douglas' bed. An outside doctor, a resident, and two interns come in to look at Alice. They all gather around her crib and chat with her mother. [The cubicle is an extremely small and public space for consulting or medical rounds. To save time, the physicians do not use the examination room thirty or forty feet down the corridor, where Alice's mother might feel freer to talk.]

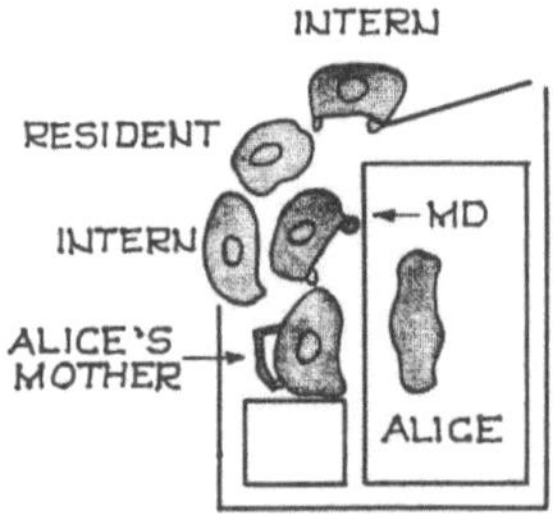


Earl comes back, having been to the playroom.

RN Benson gives him a sponge bath and changes his clothing.

*10:30* Colin has gone to receive an x-ray and returned. He is again sitting near the fish bowl, outside the nurses' station, watching for his mother to come up the elevator. [The scale of the counter surrounding the nurses' station is such that Colin cannot see into the station; and the nurses in the station can only see his IV bottle, not him. The need for an open or glazed nurses' work space is clear.]

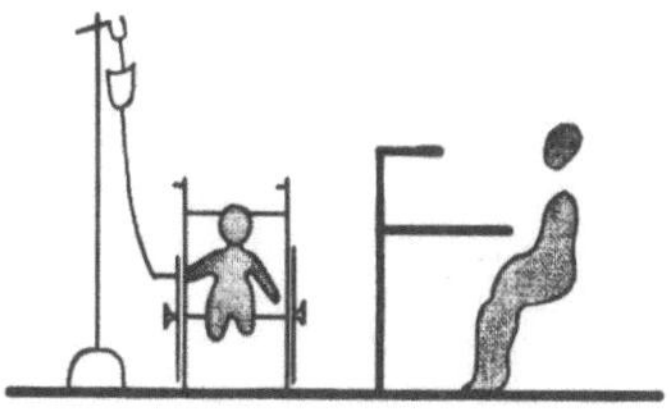

*10:45* A boy is crying in the room adjoining Room 4, adding to the general din caused by two television sets tuned to different channels. One program is a drama about a patient who is in a coma; the doctors do not know what is wrong with her. [Television seems to be used as a sort of white noise by the nursing staff. Young children seldom watch it, although their parents sometimes do. The themes of television programs are frequently medical, as here, and not necessarily appropriate for sick children. A possible solution is to develop other types of white noise.]

Four doctors are seen talking in the hallway. A fifth doctor comes in to look at Alice. [Since physicians commonly choose the corridor for an expedient conference area, thought should be given to developing private areas in the corridor. White noise surrounding alcoves off the corridor is one approach to accoustic privacy.]

A volunteer plays with Douglas, who sits in a nursery chair using an adult chair as a table. The volunteer comments that the playroom is closed for want of staff. [Again the lack of play space supervisable from the nursing area limits the richness of the child's play experience. Douglas was plainly uninterested in the type of quiet play encouraged in the crowded bed area, except when he could command the whole attention of an adult.]

*11:10* Colin is still in the corridor watching for his

mother. He stares at the elevator doors patiently and quietly.

*11:20* RN Benson draws aside the curtains between Rooms 4 and 5, then smiles at a small boy in Room 5 who can now see in to the children in Room 4. [Glazing is essential in areas for nursing young children: not only can isolated children see others, but staff can more easily supervise.]

Douglas and Earl continue to play. Brenda awakes and plays with a little toy, although still thoroughly restrained. [If the ceiling were able to accept tacks or screws, it would be possible to have mobiles or toys above Brenda's bed. As it is, boredom seems to intensify Brenda's unhappiness at being restrained.]

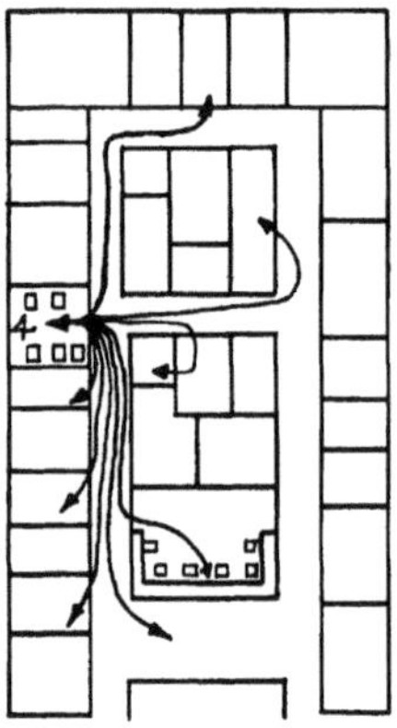


An engineer looks in for a moment and steps out, not finding any chores. A third nurse comes in with a box of tubes and bottles, talks with RN Benson, and goes out. RN Benson has several patients in Room 4 and is constantly in and out ministering to one or the other of her patients. [The five beds in Room 4 seem to constitute a subunit, with RN Benson in charge. The children know and rely on her. Her work would be simpler if she were not forced to gather supplies over the larger thirty-to-forty bed unit.]

The children do not seem to notice that the television program has again turned to medical topics, another drama about a seriously ill patient.

*11:25* Most of the nurses leave at one time for lunch. The ward is suddenly quiet. Douglas, who is curious about everything, watches a blood drawing in Room 5. A student nurse stops in to look at the children. A pediatrician comes in and talks with the student nurse about one of the children who is not taking enough fluids. Douglas listens curiously. [Again the lack of privacy for conferring is felt. In this case the student nurse has almost total responsibility for the children on Side A and must keep an eye on the children while conferring.]

*11:30* A volunteer enters and switches television stations so that the children can watch "Sesame Street," then leaves. Douglas and Earl watch, although not continuously through the program. Colin is still waiting near the nurses' station for his mother. Alice's mother is still sitting with her, looking into the mists. The student nurse comes in to do something to Douglas, who continues to watch a hairy monster learning to count to nine on "Sesame Street."

*11:45* The program holds Douglas' interest intermittently.

*11:50* The volunteer returns to collect all the toys before lunch, leaving the children in their beds without toys to await lunch, which is not served for twenty minutes. [The physical separation of play area from bed area seems to result in thinking about play as only a segment of the young child's existence, whereas it is more normal in our culture for play (and indeed learning) to provide most of a young child's activities, not a small, programmed segment of the day.]

*1:00* Douglas and Earl are napping in their beds in the darkened room. Colin is in bed, awake. He asks to have the television set on, but is told that it is nap time and television would bother the other children. He talks to himself and bothers his IV. Brenda struggles with the restraints on her arms and legs.

RN Benson turns off the lights, which lowers the light level only slightly. A mother and father can be heard talking in the next room. Many things can be seen in the hallway outside: wash pail and mop, floor polisher, x-ray viewer, supply cart, lunch gurney, extra crib, extra chair. [Strange and scary equipment is frequently stored in hospital corridors for lack of adequate storage space.]

*1:20* RN Allen comes in with medication tray and stops to say a friendly hello to the children.

*1:50* Rest period continues: Alice is crying; the others are asleep. Colin's mother comes in. She hangs up her coat on the little partition between Colin's and Douglas' beds. Colin's grandfather comes in with toys for Colin. His mother gives the grandfather her seat and sits on a nursery chair instead of taking one of the adult chairs from another child's cubicle. [Hospital visitors are often timid about moving or changing anything. Another visitor stood through an hour's visit rather than displace the package of linen that was in the visitor's chair.]

A nurse comes in and compliments Colin's behavior. His mother smiles proudly. In the background can be heard and seen a child in Room 5 being examined by two doctors. The child cries loudly, while the other child in Room 5 (a 3-year-old) looks on very seriously. Alice is still crying, almost silently, in her mist tent. She coughs occasionally. The paging system has become apparent now that the television sets are off for nap time.

*2:20* Still nap time. Everyone resting and asleep except Alice.

*2:25* RN Benson comes in with snacks and a bottle for Alice. She turns off the mist, and one is aware of the absence of a steady humming noise. She feeds the baby as Colin's mother and grandfather watch. Colin has not been awake since they arrived, and they are clearly tense, watching everything in the hallway for diversion since the television is off. The grandfather leaves.

*2:55* The children are still sleeping except Alice, who is still being burped and fed. Brenda awakes and lies quietly. RN Benson wakes up Earl so that he can eat his popsicle, which is now half melted. Earl does not enjoy being waked up and looks cross; he fusses.

3:00 Douglas has wet the bed, and the nurse talks about it loudly while changing him. Douglas does not seem to care.

## Grade School Children

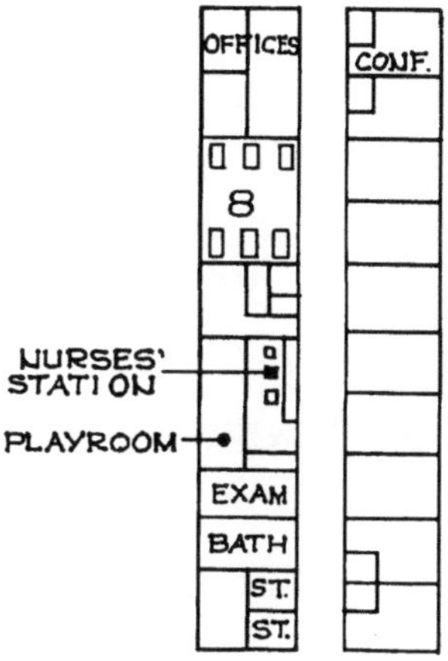


Five patients in one room, aged three to thirteen years, were observed over a period of six hours on one day and fourteen hours on the next.

Location: a community hospital, Pediatrics Unit for twenty-eight children from birth to 16 or 18 years old. Room 8, a room usually used for boys of 5–10 years. It has six beds, three or four of which are generally in use.

PERSONAE

*Allan* (9), a patient who had a herniorrhaphy yesterday.

*Bill* (5), a patient who is to have a strabotomy today.

*Charles* (7), a patient who has an infected knee.

*David* (13), a patient from a room up the hall.

*Emma* (3), a patient from across the hall.

Nursing staff: RN *Abrams*, RN *Bailey*, RN *Carlson*, RN *Dutton*, RN *Eastman*, and RN *Flores*.

Medical staff: Dr. *Adams*, Dr. *Bloom*, Dr. *Chang*, and Dr. *Duncan*.

Recreation therapist: RT *Angel*.

Maid *Alexander*.

A volunteer grandfather and several others who appear only briefly and are not named.

The nurse has awakened all the children, although Allan and Bill still seem to be dozing. The curtain has been half-opened across the window, and the room is in a grayish light.

6:50 Charles calls for the nurse. [Although there is a buzzer system (which Charles later explains in detail to his grandfather), it is seldom used. Children seem to need and rely on direct methods of communication.]

6:52 RN Abrams comes in and remonstrates with Charles. She leaves.

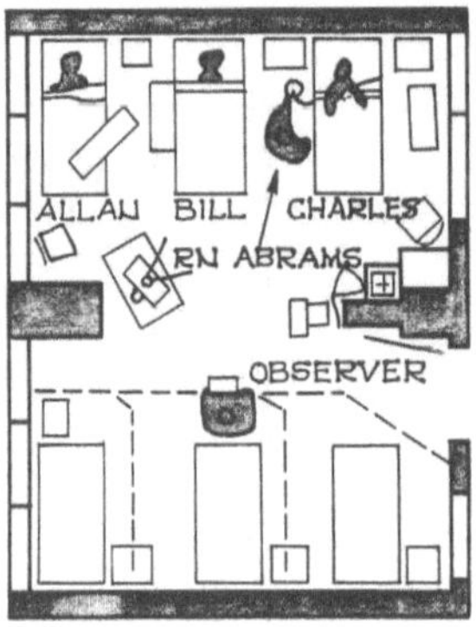


*6:55* Charles is making a crying noise. RN Abrams comes back, reproving him. RN Bailey comes with her and leaves immediately.

*7:00* Charles says, "I want my mother." RN Abrams stays in the room until he is quiet.

*7:04* Charles's phone rings. The noise wakes the others. Charles calls, "Nurse!" in alarm, then picks up the receiver. RN Abrams comes in and checks his IV. Charles carries on a murmured monosyllabic conversation on the telephone. [Charles's answering the phone is complicated by his IV apparatus: there is insufficient space to place phone, bedside table, and other objects on the side of the bed opposite the IV apparatus, although that arrangement would allow him to move more freely.]

*7:10* RN Bailey helps Allan use the urinal. This takes place in sight of the rest of the room, as she does not draw the curtains. [Allan (9) does not seem to mind the lack of privacy very much.]

*7:12* An orderly wheels a gurney into the room; he is accompanied by RN Carlson, who helps him lift sleeping Bill from his bed onto the gurney. Bill looks sleepily around. The others watch.

*7:15* The orderly wheels the gurney away. [The unexplained removal of Bill seems to be a cause for concern.]

*7:17* Charles yells for the nurse, although he still appears to be on the phone. Dr. Adams comes in to see Allan, then leaves, telling Charles he will find the nurse. A large cart is wheeled into the unit with trays on it for each patient.

*7:20* RN Carlson comes in with a breakfast tray for Charles, who stops yelling and hangs up the telephone. RN Dutton comes in with a breakfast tray for Allan. Breakfast looks usual — cereal and milk. An aide comes in with water jugs and beakers for each child; she places the jugs and beakers on the overbed table by each bed. [The overbed table, the bedside table, and almost everything in the room is on wheels, which leaves no stable place to put drinking water.]

7:22 The overhead lighting comes on outside in the corridor. RN Carlson leaves the room.

7:25 Charles starts yelling for her to come and help him eat his food. RN Dutton comes in. She helps him drink his juice. Then she goes over to Allan.

7:30 The aide, when taking Charles' water to him, tells him to stop yelling. He quiets down. Allan is asking what the time is. He shows no interest in breakfast.

7:32 Charles starts yelling for the nurse again. [Many of the children on the unit, including Charles, who is obviously upset, cannot see the nurses' station. Many times Charles seems to have called the nurse merely to see if she is still around.]

7:35 RN Eastman comes in to Charles, then she attends to Allan. She takes the breakfast trays away.

7:40 The noise level has risen considerably since waking time. Radios and television sets are on in other rooms. The loudspeaker is calling various doctors. Children in other rooms are crying or calling the nurses. Allan has found paper and crayons by his bed and is drawing.

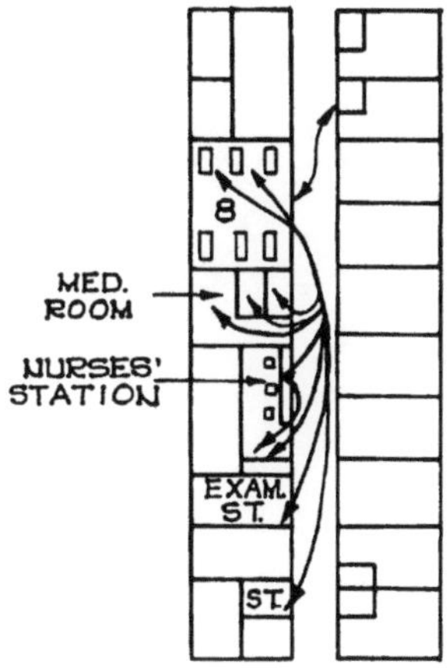


7:55 RN Dutton comes in to visit with Charles. It is her first day on the ward after a vacation, so she introduces herself to Charles and asks him several questions. Charles does not respond but looks out the window into the corridor. [RN Dutton's unrushed manner contrasts with the constant popping in and out of staff members, whose supplies, records, storage and disposal places are spread over the larger ward.]

7:57 RN Dutton goes over to Allan's bed with the same

friendliness. He complains about his operation wound. She snaps on the television set for him, turning it toward his bed.

*8:00* RN Dutton leaves the room. Dr. Adams comes back for a brief look at Allan.

*8:02* Dr. Adams leaves. RN Eastman comes in to bathe Allan. She sets him up and pulls the curtains around his bed.

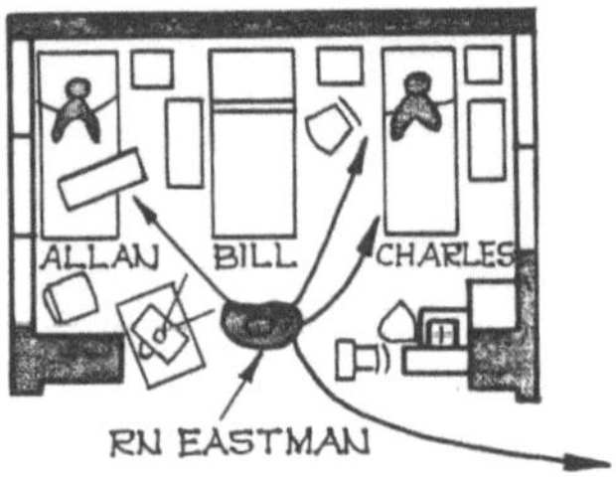


*8:05* RN Eastman goes over to Charles to give him a sponge bath. She sets him up and then goes to help Allan put on his clean pajamas.

*8:10* Charles moans and seems unable to help himself. RN Eastman goes back over to his bed to wash him, while Allan slowly eases himself out of bed. [RN Eastman's caring for Allan and Charles is complicated by the parallel bed arrangement. A more circular arrangement would allow a central space for staff, visitors, and equipment.]

*8:15* RN Eastman leaves the room and Charles starts yelling for her; she returns immediately.

*8:20* Charles watches her as she makes Allan's bed and talks to him. Charles says he wants his mother.

*8:25* RN Eastman accompanies Allan to the bathroom.

*8:26* RN Dutton comes in briefly to look for Allan. The housekeeper walks in slowly and collects the trash.

*8:28* Allan returns with RN Eastman, who then makes Charles's bed.

*8:35* RN Eastman makes Bill's bed. Allan examines his bandage with fascination while the nurse explains to him what a hernia is.

*8:37* RT Angel brings Emma, a 3-year-old patient, into the room and asks Allan and Charles if they would like to hear a story. Allan seats himself on the chair by Charles's bed, because Charles cannot get up. They all listen to a story about a little boy who was sent to the hospital for an operation. [Their grouping is awkward. In a more spacious room it would be possible to modify the furniture arrangement to arrive at a more natural seating arrangement for storytelling.]

*8:45* RN Eastman finishes making the beds and leaves the room.

*8:50* Allan complains that he is in pain. Charles seems to be asleep.

*8:55* Allan restlessly shifts in his chair. Charles moans softly to himself. There is much noise of unit activity coming from the corridor. [In general, the noise of the unit activity is reassuring: conversations, footsteps, rustling skirts, hummed tunes. At times, however, this noise includes crying and moaning which is depressing to both staff and children and could be diluted by the use of smaller units.]

*8:57* David, a 13-year-old patient, comes in carrying a Spanish comic book that he cannot read. He interrupts the recreation therapist's story to ask her for something more interesting to do. [Since David cannot be included in the cramped storytelling circle, it is hard for the play therapist to ask him to wait until the story is done.]

*9:00* RT Angel leaves to get a game from the playroom and returns with it.

*9:05* The three boys are enthusiastic about the game. A volunteer grandfather comes in and attempts to talk with David. He introduces himself to the group, but they are more interested in the game, and he leaves. [The children are very enthusiastic about the games and projects that RT Angel provides for them, but they lack even so simple a thing as a table to sit around and play the game. The overbed table which they use is awkward, too small, and the wrong height.]

*9:07* The phone by Allan's bed rings. Everyone ignores it except RT Angel, who eventually gets up, crosses the room, answers it, and hands it to Charles by stretching the cord behind Bill's bed.

*9:10* Charles talks quietly for a few minutes and hangs up. He seems to have signed out of the game, although they are still playing by his bed. He lies watching them through the bars of his cot side.

*9:15* An orderly wheels Bill in on a gurney. He is wide awake with one eye bandaged. He says he wants to sit and watch the game. [Bill and Charles, who must stay in bed, enjoy watching the others play the game.]

*9:20* RN Eastman comes to take Bill's blood pressure. RT Angel brings him a vomit bag.

*9:22* Allan leaves to go to the bathroom again. RN Eastman takes Bill's temperature.

*9:25* Allan returns from the bathroom. RN Eastman comes in to do something to Charles and then leaves. Bill dozes.

*9:27* RT Angel takes Emma, David, and Allan off to the playroom.

*9:45* Allan returns with some playthings and gets back into his bed. He is accompanied to his bedside by the volunteer grandfather.

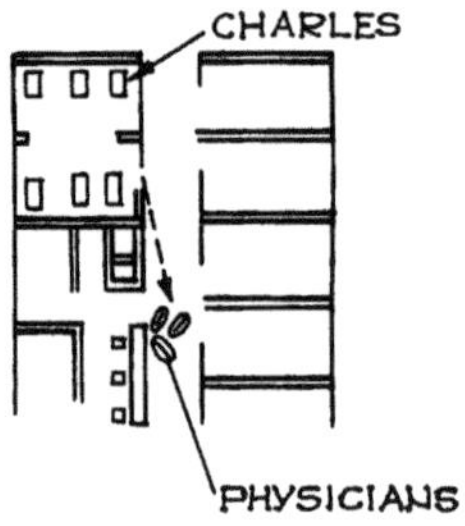


*10:00* Charles calls for the nurse again. Maid Alexander comes in.

*10:02* Three men in business suits (presumably physicians) come in and group around Charles's bed.

*10:03* Two of the men leave the room.

*10:04* RN Dutton comes in; RT Angel comes in and goes out again. The third man leaves the room, while RN Dutton stays to keep Charles company. The physicians then stand and talk at the nursing station down the corridor. [Charles can see them and presumably guess that they are talking about him; but what they are saying is inaudible and open to his imagination.]

*10:05* RN Dutton leaves. Drs. Adams, Bloom, and Chang enter to look at Charles.

*10:06* They are followed by RN Dutton and RN Eastman, and there is some discussion around Charles's bed. One doctor recommends that Charles's knee wound be bandaged.

*10:07* The three doctors hurry out of the room, followed by the two nurses. [Although Charles is scarcely pleased at being left alone in Room 8, being examined by six physicians and two nurses in the course of five minutes also seems to upset him. Some way to avoid the disturbing nature of hospital rounds must be developed. One of the things that Charles particularly notices is that many people have left him.]

On the other side of the room, the volunteer grandfather leaves Allan's bedside to talk with maid Alexander, who is vacuuming.

*10:08* The volunteer grandfather leaves the room. RN Dutton comes in with tape for Charles's leg. She is followed and helped by RN Eastman.

*10:10* RN Dutton leaves the room, but RN Eastman stays on talking with Charles. The unit clerk comes in to find out what Allan wants from the menu tomorrow.

*10:12* The unit clerk leaves the room. RN Dutton comes back into the room as Charles is moaning for his mother. Both nurses leave together.

*10:15* Charles is crying. RN Dutton returns to see Allan.

*10:17* RN Dutton leaves to get some medication for Allan as he still complains of pain. She returns immediately with RN Eastman, who comes to look after Charles.

*10:20* Dr. Duncan comes in to see Allan. He leaves.

*10:25* RT Angel brings some toys for Allan. They occupy him while she goes over to Charles, who has been asking for the "play lady." [Allan and Charles compete for RT Angel's attention, with the louder, more miserable Charles winning. The competition for the therapist's attention is intensified by the inability to place the beds in a more circular arrangement *or* to bring them into the playroom, which has a 32-inch door and cramped access through the nurses' station.]

*10:35* David comes in to find the recreation therapist and joins the game.

*10:40* Allan announces that he needs another game. RT Angel immediately leaves to find one in the playroom. Charles looks annoyed when she leaves. [The recreation therapist spends a significant proportion of her time en route between the playroom where games and craft supplies are stored and the bedrooms where many of the children must remain owing to space limitations.]

*10:42* RN Dutton comes in to adjust Charles's IV apparatus. Allan calls, "Nurse!"

*10:45* RT Angel returns, gives the game to Allan, and leaves again, as RN Dutton is still occupied with Charles's IV.

*10:47* Charles cries for the play lady. She comes back to play the game "Snakes and Ladders" with Allan.

*10:50* RT Angel repeatedly interrupts her game to comfort Charles. The pediatric psychologist enters, exchanges a few words with Charles and Allan, and leaves.

*11:05* RT Angel leaves, saying she must attend a staff meeting. Allan plays "Snakes and Ladders" with the observer. Charles receives another phone call, causing him to miss RT Angel's departure.

*11:10* RN Eastman comes and takes Allan's temperature. Another doctor comes in and looks at Charles's leg. [This is the seventh doctor who has seen Charles this morning. None has had the time to relax and be friendly, nor does the setting encourage such a practice, for the records and nursing staff with which the doctor needs contact are elsewhere on the ward.]

*11:14* RN Dutton and RN Eastman attend to Allan.

*11:15* The doctor leaves. The nurses leave, saying they are expected at a staff meeting.

*11:17* The observer is left alone with the children. Charles watches every movement as though he is afraid of being deserted by the observer as well as by everyone else.

Allan demands that the observer play endless games of "Snakes and Ladders" with him.

*11:31* RN Carlson brings in a lunch tray for Allan. He plays with his food, to the annoyance of the nurse. [Hospitalized children often eat little, except the candy and other snacks their families bring. Several strategies for encouraging better eating might be tried: provision of table and chairs to make dining a pleasant, social event, provision of a pantry/snack bar where families could prepare familiar foods (perhaps with aid from a nutritionist), and provision of cafeteria service for some meals.]

*11:32* The aide brings a lunch tray to Charles. RN Carlson and the aide leave.

*11:37* Maid Alexander comes in to clean the sink. Charles exhibits little interest in his food. He remains turned toward the hall window. [Sitting in a row, not facing one another, the boys form a very unnatural social setting for a meal, as impersonal as eating lunch at a drugstore counter.]

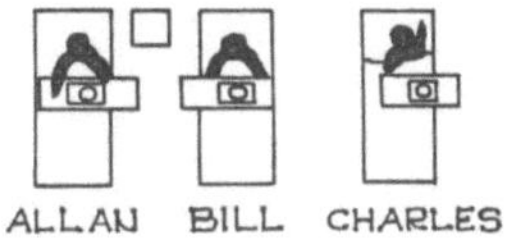


*11:45* Charles decides to eat a little and then calls the nurse. RN Flores, the head nurse, comes in and scolds him. She leaves, taking his tray.

*11:47* RN Carlson comes back and asks Allan why he has not drunk his juice. Since he put salt in it, he says it is salty. She takes his tray away.

*11:50* The aide returns in response to Charles's yells of "Nurse! nurse!" She fusses over him.

## Adolescents

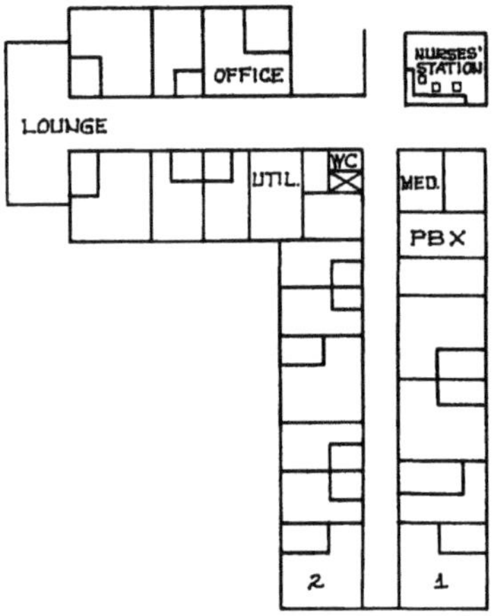


Four patients in two double rooms, aged seventeen to nineteen years, were observed over a period of fourteen hours on one day.

Location: a community hospital, Youth Unit for twenty patients from 12 to 20 years old. Rooms 1 and 2, double rooms inhabited by girls and boys respectively.

PERSONAE

*Ann* (19), a patient who has been hospitalized for several months following hip surgery.

*Beth* (19), a patient who was hospitalized the night before preparatory to minor surgery and who is normally a part-time unit clerk on this unit.

*Carl* (17), a patient who is to have a spinal operation later in the day.

*Dan* (18), a patient who is hospitalized for diagnostic tests. He has been hospitalized previously for long periods and was left lame by a spinal ailment.

Nursing staff: RN *Alberts*, RN *Brodsky*, RN *Callahan*, RN *Davis*, RN *Ernst*, and Aide *Fugii*.

Maid *Anderson*.

A unit clerk and other characters who appear briefly and are identified only by their relationship to the patients.

## Room 1

*8:20* Ann is eating breakfast lying flat on her back in traction. [Because no dining area is available, patients eat alone or in pairs in their rooms.]

Beth is taking a shower.

*8:35* RN Brodsky brings the morning newspaper and tomorrow's menu.

*8:37* RN Callahan comes in to collect Ann's breakfast tray.

*8:55* An orderly comes in to visit Beth.

*9:00* Beth seems nervous; when the orderly leaves, she goes off to "chart temps," which is one of her unit clerk jobs. [Adolescents, just like many adults, find work therapeutic when they are anxious or otherwise upset. It may be possible to reorganize nursing units to give patients useful work, such as caring for younger children, feeding each other, performing clerical jobs, or making things for other patients.]

RN Davis comes in to take Ann's leg out of traction. She leaves with the breakfast tray.

*9:10* Beth's doctor comes in looking for her. The physical therapist comes in to exercise Ann's leg.

*9:25* Beth comes back to the room with her doctor, who has found her.

*9:30* Ann and her physical therapist take crutches out into the hallway for her to practice walking with them. [What could have been an enjoyable excursion, a chance to get out of the unit altogether, cannot be because the therapists are extremely short of space and only use their exercise room for patients needing special equipment.]
Beth goes off to visit someone else. She says she is very nervous — more so about the anesthetic than about the operation.

*9:35* RN Alberts is talking with Ann. Beth comes back and goes to the bathroom.

*9:45* RN Callahan comes into each room with a tray of medication.

*9:55* The schoolteacher comes in to see Ann, and the unit clerk comes in to see Beth. [The lack of a schoolroom makes it difficult for the schoolteacher to make good use of his time; he has only a few minutes for each pupil. The patients have no feeling of *going* to school and no place to hook up by telephone, tape, or television with their home school.]

*9:58* The schoolteacher leaves, and the remaining three people chat and laugh together.

*10:00* RN Callahan brings medication for Beth and has her change into a hospital gown. The odor of medication fills the room. Ann, with her considerable hospital experience, comments on the name of the medication and the "rules" for surgery: "no jewelry, no glass eyeballs up there." [Olfactory privacy is possibly the most difficult sort of privacy to provide. A pervasive disinfectant smell provides that privacy in many hospitals, but at the cost of an unpleasant atmosphere.]

*10:02* A patient with a nurse's cap comes in to tell RN Callahan that she is wanted elsewhere. RN Brodsky comes and talks with Beth and Ann about surgery and shots.

*10:10* RN Brodsky leaves. RN Alberts enters, does something, and leaves. Beth's father stops by on his way to work in the hospital. [The necessity to entertain visitors is mentioned by patients as a chore, especially where parents are involved. Adolescents seldom sit and talk with their parents. Perhaps the hospital could offer some form of entertainment. Pool, ping-pong, and swimming are used by ambulant adolescents and their families in some hospitals.]

*10:12* RN Alberts makes Ann's bed while Ann sits uncomfortably in a chair. They chat amicably about RN Alberts' problems and seem to be close friends.

*10:25* RN Alberts leaves. Beth presses the button to move down the head of her bed because she is getting drowsy. After a few false starts, she finds the right button, and the bed head lowers with a loud screech.

*10:50* An orderly comes into the room with a gurney to pick up Beth. Everything had to be cleared off the shelf by the door in order to fold it down so that the gurney could fit in the room. [The tightness of the situation makes it troublesome to take bed patients (in bed) out on the sun porch in fine weather; in fact, it is rarely done.]

After Beth leaves, RN Callahan comes in to make 'up her bed.

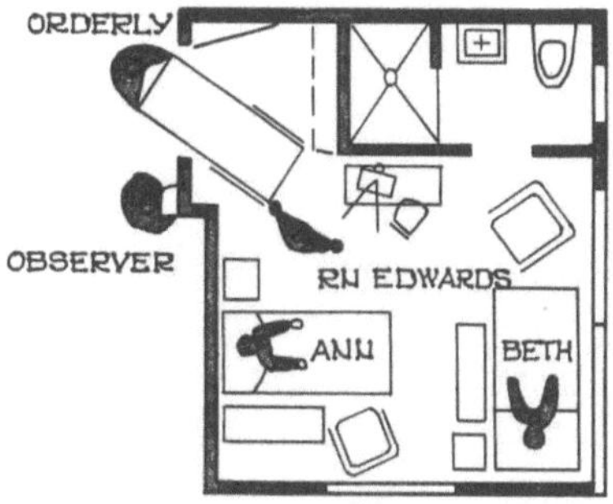

ROOM I

*10:55* Another nurse comes in to get a key from RN Callahan.

*11:00* RN Callahan leaves and returns with medication for Ann.

*11:16* RN Davis brings in a new nurse, RN Ernst, whom she introduces to Ann. They leave.

*11:20* Ann goes into the bathroom to have a shower. This is a long process for her, as she has to maneuver with a "walker."

*11:32* Maid Anderson enters with the patient in the nurse's cap, who follows her around chattering.

*1:00* A patient comes in to visit Ann.

*1:05* Another patient comes in to visit. Beth is wheeled back from surgery on a gurney. Both visitors are in wheelchairs, and they occupy the entire area inside the door because the wheelchairs are too wide to enter further into the room. Both visitors have to back out in order to let the gurney out. [If a comfortable day room were available, much of the commotion could be spared Beth, who is just coming out of anesthesia, and Ann and her friends could eat together.]

*1:07* A third patient in a wheelchair comes in, then they all back out to let the nurse leave. Beth's father enters to see her.

One of the visiting patients is going to have his lunch here, but he must wait to eat it until Ann, using the only table, has finished her lunch. [The lounge at the end of the other corridor is not enclosed enough to be comfortable as a gathering place and is too cramped for convenient use by wheelchair and gurney patients.]

*1:10* Beth's doctor and another visitor arrive for Beth, totally filling the little remaining space. Beth's doctor does a quick check on her condition. RN Ernst enters and takes Beth's blood pressure. Beth's doctor, her father, and one of her visitors leave.

## Room 2

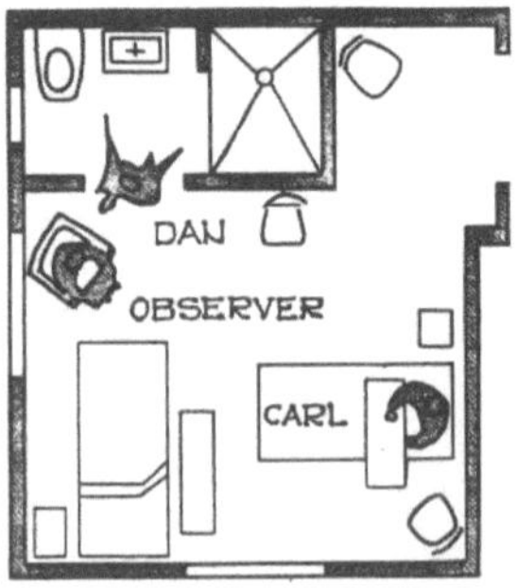


ROOM 2

*8:20* Carl is playing cards (solitaire) in lieu of breakfast. Dan is eating breakfast.

*8:25* Maid Anderson enters to clean the room, and Dan teases her. She leaves, expressing her disapproval of his teasing. RN Alberts comes in to remove Dan's breakfast tray.

*8:30* Dan gets up to go to the bathroom. He jokes rather brashly to the observer about the slowness and awkwardness of this procedure. [Adolescents are extremely sensitive about physical appearances. The fact that the observer was a woman and that there was no ambiguity whatsoever about Dan's destination must have increased his embarrassment. A bathroom opening directly off one's bed/visiting room is awkward.]

*9:10* A technician comes to get Dan for a myelogram. The gurney hardly fits into the room; Dan walks over, gets onto it, and is wheeled off.

*9:15* In leaving, Dan hands Carl his little transistor radio, which Carl turns on to a popular music station. The music can be heard down the quiet corridor. [Music, and often loud music, is an important recreational and expressive medium for adolescents, yet unless there is a special place for it in the hospital environment, it will bother some patients and may be banned.]

*9:17* RN Alberts comes in to make up Dan's bed. She does not talk to Carl, except to ask some medical questions. Carl is writing a letter.

*9:30* RN Alberts changes and tidies Carl's bed as he plays cards.

*9:35* Dan's mother and another woman arrive to visit Dan; they come into his room to wait for him. Carl has his bed curtains closed since he is washing. The women look aimless and unhappy. [Bed curtains provide only the flimsiest of barriers against the eyes, ears, and noses of others. In this case the visitors are at least as bothered as the patient.]

*9:40* RN Alberts enters and talks with Dan's visitors.

*9:45* Dan's visitors leave the room and seat themselves in the chairs at the end of the hall.

*9:58* The schoolteacher comes in and sits down next to Carl. They talk.

*10:05* The schoolteacher finishes talking with Carl and leaves.

*10:10* RN Alberts stops in to see Carl and leaves. A patient in a wheelchair pulls another patient who is lying flat on a gurney into Carl's room. They talk quietly with Carl.

*10:15* Carl's mother and sister arrive to see him, and the other patients leave.

*10:30* Dan returns from radiology on a large gurney. He is wheeled into the room, accompanied by his mother, and then the door is closed. Carl and his visitors remain, but the friend of Dan's mother, maid Anderson, and the observer wait outside the door. [Privacy is almost tabu; thus, when the technician shuts Dan's door, it is taken as a signal to worry by the maid, the visitor, and the observer.]

*10:31* The door is opened. Maid Anderson goes in to sweep the floor. Dan has been taken off the gurney and put on his bed. Dan's doctor comes in and converses softly with Dan's mother. Carl's visitors reenter. There are groans from Dan, who is obviously in great pain.

*10:40* RN Callahan comes in to see Dan.

*10:45* Dan's doctor leaves, frowning at the observer who is sitting in the corridor. There are now seven people in the room, including both patients and visitors. Carl keeps up a stream of bubbly conversation to his visitors, who are obviously concerned about his upcoming surgery and do not seem talkative. RN Callahan comes in to talk with Dan, and their conversation is listened to by the rest of the room. [Dan commented later on the difficulty of finding privacy when in pain. He definitely did not want a lot of women around when he was weakened by pain.]

Maid Anderson, whom Dan teased earlier, joins the group with quietly sympathetic words. Carl says that offering condolences is one of her favorite roles.

*10:50* Carl's relatives look on with a kind of fascinated horror, especially when Dan moans or swears aloud in pain.

*11:00* Carl's mother and sister are still standing, although they arrived forty-five minutes ago. His mother keeps her coat over her shoulders; his sister leans on the window sill. [The organization and efficiency of the hospital often make guests feel singularly out of place unless the patient is feeling well enough to entertain them, as Carl was on the morning before surgery. Rooms are seldom planned in a way that allows naturally comfortable seating patterns.]

*11:06* Carl's mother and sister decide to sit down. His

mother gets one of two easy chairs stacked by the door and puts it near Carl's bed. His sister pulls up a little wooden chair.



*11:12* RN Alberts leaves Dan, and his mother comes in.

*11:16* RN Davis stops briefly to introduce the new nurse, RN Ernst, to Carl and Dan.

*11:20* Dan is still moaning, and his mother is sitting with him. Carl's family seems to have run out of things to say. Carl, however, keeps up the conversation and makes them laugh.

*11:30* Dan puts on his light to call the nurse. He is answered by the aide, who goes to get RN Davis and the new nurse, RN Ernst.

*12:45* Dan awakes, and Carl calls to him and asks him something about the radio. RN Davis brings Dan something and half-closes his bed curtains.

*12:50* An orderly comes in with a gurney to get Carl. Maid Anderson enters. Carl's mother and sister leave. Dan is left alone with his mother and her friend.

# Appendix C
# Misery Is . . .

The following essay was written by members of the Adolescent Unit in Children's Hospital at Stanford, Palo Alto, California.

MISERY IS . . .

when you can't walk to the bathroom and you have to wait for an aide who is somewhere else;

when you're itching in a place where you can't reach it;

when the nurse wakes you up at six o'clock in the morning and makes you drink hot tea;

when you're exposed under the heat lamp and a doctor walks in and talks to you;

when you can't reach your feet and the stick that helps you get your pants over them breaks;

when the stopper on your catheter comes out and it all drains down into your shoe;

getting a nonlubricated suppository from a nurse with cold hands and long fingernails;

when you've used the bed pan and, before the nurse comes to get it, it turns over;

when the physical therapist unbuttons your pants when she grabs your belt to lift you onto the bed;

when you're being bathed and you're all uncovered and the doctors open the curtain for a consultation and ask, "Why are you lying there like *that* for?"

having a nurse say she'll find out if you can have something for your wheezing and, when she comes back, say, "No, not for two hours. How about something to drink?"

when you're feeling groovy about everything and then you see the lab man with his syringe and you notice that you're the only one in the ward and he's coming right at you;

when you didn't drink your milk at lunchtime and so you're told that you can't have your soda when you want it later on?

being nineteen years old and a boy in the hospital keeps hanging around you but he's only fourteen years old;

having the patient next to you being visited by someone who is smoking a smelly cigar while you're having an asthma attack;

when you're having an enema and an I.V. and a medical student walks in to show you his magic tricks;

when your friends are at the hospital to see you and the nurse comes in and asks, "Did you have a b.m. today?"

when your doctor is looking for you and finds you in the P.T. room right in the middle of a leg lift;

when all the kids are standing around and the nurse comes in and says very loudly that she still needs that urine specimen;

when you can't eat your lunch until the occupational therapist gets there and then it's too cold;

when you don't want to see your social worker but you don't have a class and she knows all of your hiding places;

when your friends are visiting you and the nurse comes in and asks you if you don't notice that something smells bad;

when everybody's talking about "Stupid-Dr.-What's-His-Name" and you turn around and there's "Stupid-Dr.-What's-His-Name";

when it's bedtime and you're lying bottomside up to have the red spot on it treated and one of the boys opens the curtain and says, "Goodnight," very sweetly;

not being able to turn on either side and you have a sore on your bottom;

when you're thirsty and it's a long time before anyone comes around to get you a drink;

getting up at six o'clock on "weigh day" just to find out that you've put on more weight;

when you're sitting in your wheelchair all cleaned up wearing your best dress and then discover that you're all wet because your catheter just slipped out;

having to put on your swim suit at 6:30 in the morning and you hate the swimming pool;

having a nurse say she'll find out if you can have something for your wheezing and she never comes back;

being too heavy for the scales at the Children's Hospital and you have to get weighed on the freight scale at the Stanford Hospital;

when you're going home for good and you don't want to leave all of your hospital friends but you want to go home to see all of your boyfriends.

# Notes

## 1. ALTERNATIVES TO HOSPITALIZATION

1. Robert J. Haggerty, "Present Strengths and Weaknesses in Current Systems of Comprehensive Health Services for Children and Youth," *Amer. J. Pub. Hlth.* 60, no. 4, pt. 2 (April 1970), 74.

2. René Dubos, *Man and His Environment*, Pan American Health Organization Scientific Publication no. 131 (Washington, D.C.: WHO, 1955), p. 10.

3. Roger J. Meyer and David Klein, eds., "Childhood Injuries: Approaches and Perspectives," *Supplement to Pediatrics* 44, no. 5, pt. 2 (November 1969), 791–896.

4. Katharina Dalton, "Children's Hospital Admissions and Mother's Menstruation," *Brit. Med. J.* 2 (April 4, 1970), 27–28.

5. Julius B. Richmond and Howard L. Weinberger, "Program Implications of New Knowledge Regarding the Physical, Intellectual, and Emotional Growth and Development and the Unmet Needs of Children and Youth," *Amer. J. Pub. Hlth.* 60, no. 4, pt. 2 (April 1970), 23, 28.

6. Robert A. Aldrich and Ralph J. Wedgewood, "Examination of the Changes in the United States Which Affect the Health of Children and Youth," *Amer. J. Pub. Hlth.* 60, no. 4, pt. 2 (April 1970), 9.

7. F. M. B. Allen, "Paediatrics — Past and Present," *Brit. Med. J.* 2 (December 26, 1964), 1645; Alfred White Franklin, "Paediatrics 1984," *Lancet*, January 16, 1965, p. 7377.

8. Lawrence K. Pickett, "The Hospital Environment for the Pediatric Surgical Patient," *Pediat. Clin. N. Amer.* 16, no. 3 (August 1969), 531.

9. Richmond and Weinberger, "Program Implications of New Knowledge," p. 57.

10. Count D. Gibson, Jr., "The Neighborhood Health Center: The Primary Unit of Health Care," *Amer. J. Pub. Hlth.* 58, no. 7 (July 1968), 1188–1191.

11. Harold B. Wise, E. Fuller Torrey, Adrienne McDade, Gloria Perry, and Harriet Bograd, "The Family Health Worker," *Amer. J. Pub. Hlth.* 58, no. 10 (1968), 1828–1838.

12. Dale C. Garell, "Adolescent Medicine," *Amer. J. Dis. Child.* 109 (April 1965), 314.

13. Jean A. White, "A Mobile Clinic in an Urban Area," *Nurs. Times*, November 13, 1969, p. 1458.

14. Geoffrey C. Robinson, Chandrakant P. Shah, Corinne Argue, Claire Kin-

nis, and Sydney Israels, "A Study of the Need for Alternative Types of Health Care for Children in Hospitals," *Pediatrics* 43, no. 5 (May 1969), 866; Morris Green and William E. Segar, "A New Design for Patient Care and Pediatric Education in a Children's Hospital: An Interim Report," *Pediatrics* 28, no. 5 (November 1961), 825; Frederic G. Burke, "The Pediatric Convalescence Hospital: The 30- to 90-day Extended Care Unit," *Pediatrics* 43, no. 5 (May 1969), 879.

15. M. Spagnuolo, J. Gavrin, and J. Ryan, "A Day Hospital for Children with Rheumatic Fever," *Pediatrics* 45, no. 2 (February 1970), 276.

16. "A Surgical Day Care Plan," *Hospitals* 43 (June 16, 1969), 75–76; William L. Nellis, "How a Community Hospital Holds the Line on Costs," *Hosp. Mgmt.*, November 1969, p. 32.

17. Claire F. Ryder, Pauline G. Stitt, and William F. Elkin, "Home Health Services — Past, Present, Future," *Amer. J. Pub. Hlth.* 59, no. 9 (September 1969), 1720.

18. Medical procedures that have been carried out in the home include urine collection, hematology tests, lumbar puncture, subdural tap, duodenal intubation, esophageal catheter, and electrocardiography. Therapeutic procedures that have been carried out at home include physiotherapy, mist tent, oxygen administration, incision of abscess, dressing changes, limb traction, parenteral fluid administration, blood transfusion, and fluids per rectum. It may be more convenient to carry out some of these procedures (such as lumbar puncture, subdural tap, abscess incision, and intravenous feeding), in the outpatient department and then return the patient to his home. A. B. Bergman, H. Shrand, and T. E. Oppé, "A Pediatric Home Care Program in London — Ten Years' Experience," *Pediatrics* 36, no. 3, pt. 1 (September 1965), 320.

19. K. C. Finkel and Shirley E. Pitt, "Pediatric Home Care Program: Review of Two and a Half Years' Experience at the Children's Hospital of Winnepeg," *Canad. Med. Ass. J.* 98 (January 20, 1968), 162.

20. M. Jeanette Juntti, "Problem Solving in Arranging for Comprehensive Home Care," *Nurs. Forum* 8, no. 1 (1969), 103.

## 2. THE HOSPITAL ENVIRONMENT AND THE COMMUNITY

1. Frederic W. Ilfeld, Jr., and Erich Lindemann, "Professional and Community: Pathways Toward Trust," Paper presented to the American Psychiatric Association, Washington, D.C., May 1971; Anselm Straus, ed., *Where Medicine Fails* (Chicago: Aldine, 1970).

2. H. Jack Geiger, "Of the Poor, by the Poor, or for the Poor: The Mental Health Implications of Social Control of Poverty Programs," *Psychiat. Res. Rep. Amer. Psychiat. Ass.* 21 (January 1967), 55–65.

3. G. L. Tischler, "The Effect of Consumer Control upon the Delivery of Service," *Am. J. Ortho. Psychiat.* 40, no. 2 (March 1970), 275– 276.

4. Panel discussion at the Fifth Annual Conference of the American Association for Child Care in Hospitals, San Francisco, April 1970.

5. Lucy Muldrow, RN, Clinic Coordinator, Berkeley Health Department, Berkeley, Cal., communication to authors, February 1970.

6. Mayer Spivack, "Sensory Distortions in Tunnels and Corridors," *Hosp. and Commun. Psychiat.*, January 1967, pp. 24–30.

## 3. ENVIRONMENTS FOR INFANTS

1. John Bowlby, "The Nature of the Child's Tie to His Mother," *Int. J. Psycho-Anal.* 39 (1958), p. 350.

2. Harry Bakwin, "Loneliness in Infants," *Amer. J. Dis. Child* 63 (January 1942), 30–40; John Bowlby, *Child Care and the Growth of Love* (Baltimore: Penguin Books, 1965); William Goldfarb, "Effects of Psychological Deprivations in Infancy and Subsequent Stimulation," *Amer. J. Psychiat.* 102 (1945), 18; René A. Spitz, "Hospitalism: An Inquiry into the Genesis of Psychiatric Conditions in Early Childhood," in *Psychoanalytic Study of the Child* (New York: International Universities Press, 1945), I, 53–74.

3. Peter H. Wolff and Richard I. Feinbloom, "Critical Periods and Cognitive Development in the First 2 Years," *Pediatrics* 44 (1969), 999.

4. Catherine Landreth, *Early Childhood Behavior and Learning* (New York: Alfred A. Knopf, 1967), p. 106.

5. Myriam David and Geneviève Appell, "A Study of Nursing Care and Nurse-Infant Interaction," in *Determinants of Infant Behavior*, ed. B. M. Foss (London: Methuen, 1961), pp. 121–135.

6. John Bowlby, *Maternal Care and Mental Health*, WHO Monograph Series no. 2 (Geneva, 1952).

7. Spitz, "Hospitalism," pp. 53–74.

8. Goldfarb, "Effects of Psychological Deprivations," p. 18.

9. Harriet Lange Rheingold, "The Modification of Social Responsiveness in Institutional Babies," Society for Research in Child Development Monograph no. 21, ser. 63, pt. 2 (1965).

10. Dane G. Prugh, "Emotional Aspects of the Hospitalization of Children," in *Red Is the Color of Hurting: Planning for Children in the Hospital*, ed. Milton F. Shore (Bethesda: NIMH, 1965), available from Superintendent of Documents, Washington, D.C.

11. John Bowlby, "The Nature of the Child's Tie," p. 350.

12. H. R. Schaffer and W. M. Callender, "Psychologic Effects of Hospitalization in Infancy," *Pediatrics* 24 (1959), 528–539.

13. Bowlby, *Child Care*, pp. 178–179.

14. Urie Bronfenbrenner, *Two Worlds of Childhood* (New York: Russell Sage Foundation, 1970), p. 17.

15. Melford E. Spiro, *Kibbutz: Venture in Utopia* (Cambridge, Mass.: Harvard University Press, 1956), p. 131.

16. Leon J. Yarrow, "Separation from Parents during Early Childhood," in *Review of Child Development Research*, ed. M. L. Hoffman and L. W. Hoffman (New York: Russell Sage Foundation, 1964), pp. 89–103; Louise Sandler and Barbara Torpie, "Improvement of Residential Care of Infants and Children from Birth to Age 3," *Arch. Environ. Hlth.* 17 (July 1968), 80.

17. Discussions with nursing staff at Children's Hospital at Stanford, where children from birth to six years share a unit, reinforce these points.

18. Harold Stuart and Dane G. Prugh, *The Healthy Child* (Cambridge, Mass.: Harvard University Press, 1960), p. 252.

19. Harlow and Zimmerman in experiments on newborn monkeys indicate that one important function of the mother, in addition to feeding, is to provide tactile stimulation or "comfort contact." Harry F. Harlow and Robert R. Zim-

merman, "Affectional Responses in the Infant Monkey," *Science* 130, no. 3373 (1959), 421–432.

20. Emma N. Plank, *Working with Children in Hospitals: A Guide for the Professional Team* (Cleveland: The Press of Western Reserve University, 1962), p. 35.

21. Bronfenbrenner, *Two Worlds*, p. 17.

22. Susanna Millar, *The Psychology of Play* (Baltimore: Penguin Books, 1968), p. 105.

23. Millar, *The Psychology of Play*, p. 104.

24. Robert L. Frantz, "The Origin of Form Perception," *Sci. Amer.* 204, no. 5 (May 1961), 66–72.

## 4. ENVIRONMENTS FOR TODDLERS AND PRESCHOOLERS

1. Catherine Landreth, *Early Childhood: Behavior and Learning* (New York: Alfred A. Knopf, 1967), p. 331.

2. Dane G. Prugh, "Emotional Aspects of the Hospitalization of Children," in *Red is the Color of Hurting: Planning for Children in the Hospital*, ed. Milton F. Shore (Bethesda: NIMH, 1965), available from Superintendent of Documents, Washington, D.C., pp. 20–21.

3. Herb Caen, *San Francisco Chronicle*, September 16, 1970, p. 31.

4. Kaiser Foundation hospitals have been developed on this principle.

5. George H. Lowrey, "The Problem of Hospital Accidents to Children," *Pediatrics* 32, no. 6 (December 1963), 1064–1065.

6. Gladys S. Benz, "Safety — A Component of Child Care," *Pediatric Nursing*, 5th ed. (St. Louis: C. V. Mosby, 1964), pp. 93–103.

7. Marshall B. Kreidberg, Hermann H. Field, Delbert Highlands, and Donald A. Kennedy with Geneva Katz, "Problems of Pediatric Hospital Design," multilith, The Boston Floating Hospital for Infants and Children, Tufts-New England Medical Center, Boston (November 30, 1965), p. 138.

8. Kreidberg et al., "Problems of Pediatric Hospital Design," p. 139.

9. Erving Goffman, *Asylums: Essays on the Social Situations of Mental Patients and Other Inmates* (Garden City: Doubleday, 1961), pp. 14–48.

10. Catherine Landreth, *Education of the Young Child: A Nursery School Manual* (New York: John Wiley, 1942), p. 78.

11. Benjamin Spock, *Baby and Child Care*, rev. ed. (New York: Pocket Books, 1968), pp. 249–264.

12. Spock, *Baby and Child Care*, p. 262.

13. Rhoda Kellogg, *Nursery School Guide: Theory and Practice for Teachers and Parents* (Boston: Houghton Mifflin, 1949), p. 15.

14. Selma H. Fraiberg, *The Magic Years: Understanding and Handling the Problems of Early Childhood* (New York: Charles Scribner's, 1959), p. 94.

15. Hugh Jolly, "Play Is Work," *Lancet*, August 30, 1969, pp. 487–488.

16. Landreth, *Early Childhood*, p. 117.

17. Richard Dattner, *Design for Play* (New York: Van Nostrand Reinhold, 1969), pp. 27–28.

18. C. Th. Sørensen, Preface to Marjorie Allen, *Planning for Play* (Cambridge, Mass.: MIT Press, 1968), p. 9.

19. American Academy of Pediatrics, *Care of Children in Hospitals* (Evanston, Ill.: AAP, 1960), p. 27.

20. Division for Architectural Studies of the Nuffield Foundation, *Children in Hospital: Studies in Planning* (London: Oxford University Press, 1963), p. 93.

21. Kellogg, *Nursery School Guide*, pp. 15–16.

22. Landreth, *Education of the Young Child*, p. 107.

23. Great Britain, Ministry of Health, Central Health Services Council, *The Welfare of Children in Hospital*, Report of the Committee, Sir Harry Platt, Chairman (London: Her Majesty's Stationary Office, 1959), p. 9.

24. Nuffield Foundation, *Children in Hospital*, p. 93.

25. Landreth, *Early Childhood*, p. 176.

26. Landreth, *Early Childhood*, p. 163.

27. Susanna Millar, *The Psychology of Play* (Baltimore: Penguin Books, 1968), p. 112.

28. Landreth, *Education of the Young Child*, p. 201.

29. Mayer Spivack, "Listen, Hide, Build, Sing, and Dig," *Landscape Architecture* 59, no. 4 (July 1969), 292.

30. Ruth E. Hartley, Lawrence K. Frank, and Robert M. Goldenstein, *Understanding Children's Play* (New York: Columbia University Press, 1952), p. 126.

31. Landreth, *Education of the Young Child*, p. 25.

## 5. ENVIRONMENTS FOR GRADE SCHOOL CHILDREN

1. Ernest H. Watson and George H. Lowrey, *Growth and Development of Children*, 5th ed. (Chicago: Year Book Medical Publishers, 1967), p. 187.

2. Jean Piaget and Bärbel Inhelder, *The Psychology of the Child*, trans. Helen Weaver (New York: Basic Books, 1969), pp. 92–129.

3. Mollie S. Smart and Russell C. Smart, *Children: Development and Relationships* (New York: Macmillan, 1967), p. 344.

4. Norman Livson and Harvey Peskin, "Prediction of Adult Psychological Health in a Longitudinal Study," *J. Abnorm. Soc. Psychol.* 72, no. 6 (1967), 509–518.

5. Lucie Jessner, "Some Observations on Children Hospitalized during Latency," in *Dynamic Psychopathology in Childhood*, ed. Lucie Jessner and Eleanor Pavenstedt (New York: Grune & Stratton, 1959), pp. 257–268.

6. Dane G. Prugh, Elizabeth M. Staub, Harriet H. Sands, Ruth M. Kirschbaum, and Ellenora A. Lenihan, "A Study of the Emotional Reactions of Children and Families to Hospitalization and Illness," *Amer. J. Orthopsychiat.* 23, no. 1 (January 1953), 70–106.

7. Martha L. Adams and Dorothy C. Berman, "The Hospital Through a Child's Eyes," *Children* 12, no. 3 (May–June 1965), 102.

8. "Television Goes to School," *Hosp. Mgmt.* 101 (February 1966), 40–42.

9. Frances A. Mullen, "Staffing Special Education in 34 Large Cities," *J. Excep. Child.* 25, no. 4 (December 1958), 167.

10. Hedley G Dimock, *The Child in Hospital: A Study of His Emotional and Social Well-Being* (Philadelphia: F. A. Davis, 1960), pp. 102–109.

11. W. B. Schoenbohm, *Planning and Operating Facilities for Crippled Children* (Springfield, Ill.: Charles C Thomas, 1962), p. 39.

12. For a description of an adventure playground for hospitalized children,

see Marjorie Allen, *Planning for Play* (Cambridge, Mass.: MIT Press, 1968), pp. 124–125.

13. Mayer Spivack, "Listen, Hide, Build, Sing, and Dig," *Landscape Architecture* 59, no. 4 (July 1969), 292.

14. Donald Brault, "Environment for Learning: Classroom, Gymnasium and Playground," in *Physical Education for Children's Healthful Living*, ed. Margaret Rasmussen, Association for Childhood Education International Bulletin no. 23-A (Washington, D.C., 1968), p. 58.

15. R. D. Laing, *Politics of Experience* (New York: Pantheon Books, 1967).

16. "Report to Governor of California on the Migrant Master Plan," mimeo., Governor's Office, Sacramento, Cal., 1966.

17. Christopher Alexander, "From a Set of Forces to a Form," in *The Manmade Object*, ed. Gyorgy Kepes, Vision and Value Series (New York: George Braziller, 1966), pp. 105–107.

18. Smart and Smart, *Children*, pp. 422–423.

19. Benjamin Spock and Marion O. Lerrigo, *Caring for Your Disabled Child* (New York: Macmillan, 1965), pp. 164–174.

20. Emma N. Plank, *Working with Children in Hospitals: A Guide for the Professional Team* (Cleveland: The Press of Western Reserve University, 1962), p. 9.

## 6. ENVIRONMENTS FOR ADOLESCENTS

1. Leon Eisenberg, "A Developmental Approach to Adolescence," *Children* 12, no. 4 (July–August 1965), pp. 131–135; Sheldon D. Glass, "The Adolescent Patient: An Overview," *Maryland State Med. J.*, April 1969, p. 48.

2. William G. Bach, "Teenage Patients," *Hospitals* 44 (January 16, 1970), pp. 51–53.

3. Kenneth A. Wells, "The Adolescents," *Texas Med.* 65 (March 1969), 60–65.

4. U.S., Bureau of the Census, *Statistical Abstract of the United States: 1970* (Washington, D.C., 1970), p. 10; Dale C. Garell, "Adolescent Medicine: A Survey in the United States and Canada," *Amer. J. Dis. Child.* 109 (April 1965), p. 314.

5. James H. Winchester, "Teenagers Are No Longer Hospital Misfits," *Mod. Hosp.*, September 1969, pp. 144–148.

6. Dale C. Garell to authors.

7. Winchester, "Teenagers," p. 144.

8. See also C. Andrew Rigg and Rona C. Fisher, "The Ideal Adolescent Ward," Paper presented at the Society for Adolescent Medicine, Coventry, England, July 1970.

9. Dr. Joseph P. Michelson, organizer of the Adolescent Clinic at Jewish Hospital, Brooklyn, N.Y., quoted in Winchester, "Teenagers," p. 148.

10. Rigg and Fisher, "The Ideal Adolescent Ward," pp. 2–4.

11. Laurence Finberg, "Montefiore Plans Full Floor For Teen-Agers," *Mod. Hosp.* 108, no. 3 (March 1967), 128–129.

12. Bach, "Teenage Patients," p. 51.

13. Mary Lou Byers, "The Hospitalized Adolescent," *Nurs. Outlook* 15, no. 8 (August 1967), 32–34.

14. Dane G. Prugh, "Emotional Aspects of the Hospitalization of Children,"

in *Red Is the Color of Hurting: Planning for Children in the Hospital*, ed. Milton F. Shore (Bethesda: NIMH, 1965), available from Superintendent of Documents, Washington, D.C., p. 22; Thesi Bergmann, *Children in the Hospital* (New York: International Universities Press, 1965).

15. See Edward T. Hall, *The Hidden Dimension* (Garden City, N.Y.: Doubleday, 1966), as well as works by John B. Calhoun, Robert Ardrey, Nikolaas Tinbergen, C. R. Carpenter, and Konrad Lorenz.

16. Russell Barton, "The Patient's Personal Territory," *Hosp. and Commun. Psychiat.* 17, no. 2 (November 1966), 336.

17. An essay on misery written by patients in the Adolescent Unit of Children's Hospital at Stanford was primarily concerned with the lack of personal privacy. See Appendix C.

18. Bach, "Teenage Patients," pp. 51–53.

19. Selwyn Goldsmith, *Designing for the Disabled*, 2nd ed. (New York: McGraw-Hill, 1967), p. 75.

20. For detailed instructions on the installation of hoists, grab bars, ceiling eye bolts, and other aids for the weak or handicapped, see Goldsmith, *Designing for the Disabled.*

21. Bach, "Teenage Patients," p. 51.

22. Robert Goodman, "Liberated Zone: An Evolving Learning Space," *Harv. Ed. Rev.* 39, no. 4 (1969), 90–91.

23. Robert Sommer, *Personal Space: The Behavioral Basis of Design* (Englewood Cliffs, N.J.: Prentice-Hall, 1969), p. 85.

## 7. ENVIRONMENTS FOR FAMILY PARTICIPATION

1. Edward A. Mason, "The Hospitalized Child — His Emotional Needs," *New Eng. J. Med.* 272 (February 25, 1965), 406–414.

2. Great Britain, Ministry of Health, Central Health Services Council, *The Welfare of Children in Hospital*, Report of the Committee, Sir Harry Platt, Chairman (London: Her Majesty's Stationary Office, 1959), p. 38.

3. "A large number of publications have attempted to conceptualize the reactions of children and families to the experience of a child's illness and hospitalization. With regard to short-term hospitalization, the early observations of Bakwin (1942), Bakwin and Bakwin (1942), E. Jackson (1942), Levy (1945), Senn (1945), Jensen and Comly (1948), and Langford (1948) should be mentioned, among others. These were followed by the studies of Robertson (1952 and 1953) and Anna Freud (1951) on young children, of Prugh and his associates on preschool and school-age children (1953), and of Schaffer and Callender (1959) on infants. Jessner and her colleagues (1952) as well as Faust and his coworkers (1952) studied the reactions of children to tonsillectomy, as Vaughan (1957) did the same in relation to eye operations. The work of Spitz and Wolfe (1946), Roudinesco-Aubry (1952), and Heinecke (1956) on the reactions of infants and young children to separation from their parents has also had an important influence on the approach to hospitalization of young children. Bowlby's studies (1952) have illuminated the problems in long-term hospitalization or institutionalization of children, as has the work of Provence and Coleman (1962) and other investigators . . . these studies and the recent observations of Bergman (1965) and others (Geist, 1965) . . . present a

framework for viewing the hospitalization experience in children." Dane G. Prugh, "Emotional Aspects of the Hospitalization of Children, in *Red Is the Color of Hurting: Planning for Children in the Hospital*, ed. Milton F. Shore (Bethesda: NIMH, 1965), available from Superintendent of Documents, Washington, D.C., p. 19.

4. Albert J. Ochsner and Meyer J. Sturm, *The Organization, Construction and Management of Hospitals* (Chicago: Cleveland Press, 1907), p. 517.

5. In answer to a questionnaire, 151 general hospitals with over 350 beds indicated that only 21 of their pediatric departments had facilities for parents to live in. Of 91 children's hospitals in the United States and Canada responding to a questionnaire, 21 provided facilities for mothers living in, at costs ranging from no charge to $5.00 per day. Robert H. Dombro, Appendix B, in *The Hospitalized Child and His Family*, ed. J. Alex Haller, Jr. (Baltimore: The Johns Hopkins Press, 1967), p. 114.

6. Arthur D. Colman, "Territoriality in Man: A Comparison of Behavior in Home and Hospital," *Amer. J. Orthopsychiat.* 38 (1968), 464.

7. S. R. Meadow, "No, Thanks; I'd Rather Stay at Home," *Brit. Med. J.* 2, no. 5412 (September 26, 1964), 813.

8. B. D. Morgan, "Mothers in Hospital: The Nurses' Viewpoint," *Lancet*, July 1, 1967, pp. 38–39.

9. Dorothy C. Berman, "Pediatric Nurses as Mothers See Them," *Amer. J. Nurs.* 66, no. 11 (November 1966), 2429–2431.

10. Frederick W. Seidl, "Pediatric Nursing Personnel and Parent Participation: A Study in Attitudes," *Nurs. Res.* 18, no. 1 (January–February 1969), 43. Seidl shows that nurses' aides hold more accepting attitudes toward parent participation than do practical nurses.

11. William Bruce Cameron, *Informal Sociology* (New York: Random House, 1963), p. 60.

12. John Elderkin Bell, *The Family in the Hospital: Lessons from Developing Countries*, Public Health Service Publication no. 1933 (Chevy Chase, Md.: NIMH, 1969).

13. Vernon L. James, Jr., and Warren E. Wheeler, "The Care-by-Parent Unit," *Pediatrics* 43, no. 4, pt. 1 (April 1969), 488.

14. Dorothy L. Merrow and Betty Sue Johnson, "Perceptions of the Mother's Role with Her Hospitalized Child," *Nurs. Res.* 17, no. 2 (March–April 1968), 155.

15. Trude R. Aufhauser, "Parent Participation in Hospital Care of Children," *Nurs. Outlook*, January 1967, p. 40; Maryrose Condon and Carolyn Peters, "Family Participation Unit," *Amer. J. Nurs.* 68, no. 3 (March 1968), 504–507; Stanley L. Englebardt, "Care-by-Parent Relieves Emotional Strain on Children, Financial Strain on Parents," *Mod. Hosp.*, December 1969, pp. 94–97; "Family Program in Children's Cancer Unit," *Hospitals* 39 (March 16, 1965), 66–69; Morris Green, "A New Arrangement for Hospital Services: The Parent-Care Pavilion," *Pediatrics* 43, no. 4, pt. 1 (April 1969), 486–487; Geneva Katz, "Mothers Help Care for Sick Children in Experimental Unit," *Hospitals* 38, no. 13 (July 1, 1964), 38; Ellen Leman, "Mothers Make Effective Aides at Hunterdon Medical Center," *Hosp. Topics*, October 1966, p. 95; Margarita Meagher, "Family-Centered Pediatrics," *Hospital Progr.*, November 1967, pp. 100–102; Marino Ortolani, "Mothers in Residence: Mothers as Nursing Attendants in a Children's Hospital in Italy," *Clin. Pediat.* 9, no. 1 (January 1970), 63–64;

Olivia Rousseau, "Mothers Do Help in Pediatrics," *Amer. J. Nurs.*, April 1967, p. 798; Joanne Shope, "Parental Involvement Program," *Nurs. Outlook*, April 1970, pp. 32–34.

16. "In the fiscal year July 1, 1966, through June 30, 1967, the comparative cost for operation of the two units, including meals, is as follows: Care-by-Parent Unit — 2,932 patient days at $19.76 per day. The acute, general pediatric ward — 12,667 patient days at $33.93 per patient day. These figures do not reflect any cost incurred for drugs, laboratory determinations, x-rays, and so forth . . . The hospital administration is satisfied that Care-by-Parent Unit costs 40% less than the acute, general pediatric ward." James and Wheeler, "The Care-by-Parent Unit," pp. 492–493.

17. Shope, "Parental Involvement Program," p. 33.

18. D. J. Brain and Inga Maclay, "Controlled Study of Mothers and Children in Hospital," *Brit. Med. J.* 1, no. 5587 (February 3, 1968), 278; Meadow, "No, Thanks; I'd Rather Stay at Home," pp. 813–814; Meadow, "The Captive Mother," *Arch. Dis. Childh.* 44 (1969), 363.

19. Seidl, "Pediatric Nursing Personnel," p. 40.

20. Meadow, "The Captive Mother," p. 363.

## 8. ENVIRONMENTS FOR STAFF

1. Hedley G. Dimock, *The Child in Hospital: A Study of His Emotional and Social Well-Being* (Philadelphia: F. A. Davis, 1960), p. 165.

2. Samuel W. Bloom, *The Doctor and His Patient: A Sociological Interpretation* (New York: The Free Press, 1965), p. 171.

3. Dimock, *The Child in Hospital*, p. 165.

4. Christopher Alexander, Sara Ishikawa, and Murray Silverstein, *A Pattern Language Which Generates Multi-Service Centers* (Berkeley, Cal.: Center for Environmental Structure, 1968), pp. 265–269.

5. Esther Lucile Brown, *Newer Dimensions of Patient Care*, Pt. 2, *Improving Staff Motivation and Competence in the General Hospital* (New York: Russell Sage Foundation, 1962), p. 13.

6. Robert J. Pelletier and John D. Thompson, "Yale Index Measures Design Efficiency," *Mod. Hosp.* 95 (November 1960), 73–77.

7. Brown, *Newer Dimensions*, Pt. 2, p. 17.

8. Herman M. Somers and Anne R. Somers, *Medicare and the Hospitals: Issues and Prospects* (Washington, D.C.: The Brookings Institution, 1967), p. 114.

9. National Commission for the Study of Nursing and Nursing Education, "Summary Report on Recommendations," *Amer. J. Nurs.* 70, no. 2 (February 1970), 281.

10. Somers and Somers, *Medicare and the Hospitals*, pp. 116–117, 122–123.

11. Isabel Menzies describes the system of doing a few tasks for many patients, often thirty or more, as a technique for avoiding involvement with patients which results in anxiety. Menzies, "A Case Study of Social Systems as a Defense Against Anxiety: A Report of a Study of the Nursing Service of a General Hospital," *Hum. Relat.* 13, no. 2 (1960), 101–109 (quoted in Brown, *Newer Dimensions*, Pt. 2).

12. Brown, *Newer Dimensions*, Pt. 2, pp. 71–72. See also "Nurses, Nursing, and the ANA," *Amer. J. Nurs.* 70, no. 4 (April 1970), 808–815.

13. Brown, *Newer Dimensions*, Pt. 2, p. 25.

14. Edward T. Hall, *The Hidden Dimension* (Garden City, N.Y.: Doubleday, 1966).

15. Brown, *Newer Dimensions*, Pt. 2, pp. 40–44.

16. Somers and Somers, *Medicare and the Hospital*, pp. 103, 104.

17. C. Rufus Rorem, *Physician's Private Offices at Hospitals*, American Hospital Association Monograph no. 5 (Chicago, 1959), p. 10.

18. Dimock, *The Child in Hospital*, p. 75.

9. THE PEDIATRIC NURSING UNIT

1. Great Britain, Ministry of Health, Central Health Services Council, *The Welfare of Children in Hospital*, Report of the Committee, Sir Harry Platt, Chairman (London: Her Majesty's Stationary Office, 1959), p. 9.

2. American Academy of Pediatrics, *Care of Children in Hospitals* (Evanston, Ill.: AAP, 1960), p. 21.

3. Marshall B. Kreidberg, Hermann H. Field, Delbert Highlands, and Donald A. Kennedy with Geneva Katz, "Problems of Pediatric Hospital Design," multilith, The Boston Floating Hospital for Infants and Children, Tufts-New England Medical Center, Boston (November 30, 1965), p. 28.

4. Emma N. Plank, *Working with Children in Hospitals: A Guide for the Professional Team* (Cleveland: The Press of Western Reserve University, 1962).

5. Division for Architectural Studies of the Nuffield Foundation, *Children in Hospital: Studies in Planning* (London: Oxford University Press, 1963), p. 87.

6. Plank, *Working with Children in Hospitals*, pp. 9, 13.

# Index

Bei Fragen zur Produktsicherheit wenden Sie sich bitte an:
If you have any questions regarding product safety,
please contact:

Walter de Gruyter GmbH
Genthiner Straße 13
10785 Berlin
productsafety@degruyterbrill.com